STRUGGLE FOR HEALTH

STRUGGLE FOR HEALTH

A Case Study of Malnutrition and Ill-Health among South Indian Tribals

STUART GILLESPIE

CONCEPT PUBLISHING COMPANY, NEW DELHI-110059

ISBN 81-7022-463-2

First Published 1993

Published and Printed by
Ashok Kumar Mittal
Concept Publishing Company
A/15-16, Commercial Block, Mohan Garden
NEW DELHI-110059

Lasertypeset by
Microtech Advance Printing Systems (Pvt.) Ltd.
H-13, Bali Nagar
NEW DELHI-110015

To Lindsay

TABLE OF CONTENTS

1

INTRODUCTION

The aim of this research is to build a coherent and interdisciplinary longitudinal analysis of the social and economic processes with which disease and malnutrition amongst children are associated. The environmental context is a set of small tribal villages in a remote part of Andhra Pradesh, South India.

The aetiology of malnutrition is multifaceted, involving interactions between social, economic and political forces, household level factors, disease vectors and individual characteristics. Research concentrating on single variables is limited by conditions which often are neither explicitly acknowledged nor fulfilled. Many studies are *ad hoc* in nature and lacking in theoretical contextualisation. Despite cogent arguments for a more comprehensive multidisciplinary approach to nutrition studies (Schofield 1974; Chambers 1983; Timmer *et al.* 1983) few of this kind have been undertaken on the sub-continent.

1.1 THE AETIOLOGY OF MALNUTRITION: A REVIEW

It has been established that malnutrition is not randomly distributed within a given population, but is simultaneously an outcome and cause of poverty (Rawson and Valverde 1976; Valverde *et al.* 1977; Levinson 1978; Tripp 1981; Sukhatme 1981; UNICEF 1981; Lipton 1983; Nabarro 1984; Martorell *et al.* 1984). The ability of a household to command adequate food resources - through self-production or market transactions - is primarily dependent upon assets and/or income. In agrarian societies, land ownership has been shown to be a sensitive indicator of wealth, and studies have indicated that malnutrition is associated with the lack of such a productive asset (Rawson and Valverde 1976; Valverde *et al.* 1977; Tripp 1981; Nabarro 1984; Martorell *et al.* 1984) and/or low effective income (Wray and Aguirre 1969; Bairagi 1980; Lipton 1983; Murrillo 1983; Becker *et al.* 1986).

However, although many investigators have found it possible to correlate socio-economic status and child growth at the community level, in some cases (Plattner 1974; Taylor *et al.* 1978; Stinson 1983; Ryan *et al.* 1984; Bhuiya *et al.*,1986), this has not been found, leading to the suggestion that there may be insufficient economic inequality in poor communities for socio-economic status to affect child growth.

Poverty may be exacerbated at certain times of the year through the effect of seasonality on the availability of food and income (Raikes 1981). Seasonality in labour demand may have a considerable effect on child nutritional status, particularly where changes in patterns of maternal time allocation and adverse intra-household food allocation coincide with periods of increased disease incidence (Longhurst and Payne 1979). The tendency in India for births to peak during or just before a period of intense female work input may lead to an increased risk of infant and child mortality (Crookes and Dyson 1981) and/or have an adverse effect on the efficacy of breast-feeding (Rajagopalan *et al.* 1981). Gambian studies have shown the adverse nutritional consequences for the child of the mother's decision to initiate weaning abruptly at times of peak demand for family female labour (Thompson and Rahaman 1967).

Female participation in waged work may have countervailing effects on child nutrition. Mothers' economic participation has been shown in Ghana, for example, to lead to improved child nutritional status through increasing income and effective demand for food (Tripp 1981). In the Philippines, however, the net effect of maternal labour force participation was detrimental to child nutritional status, as inadequate time was devoted to child care and feeding (Popkin 1980).

Within the household unit, demographic factors can exert an effect on child nutrition. Child nutritional status has been shown to be significantly lower for children from large families (Mukherjee and Sethna 1972; Grewal *et al.* 1973; Gupta and Srivastava 1977; Levinson 1978; Wolfe and Behrman 1982; Aguillon *et al.* 1985), with short birth intervals (Mudkhedkar and Shah 1976), and of high birth order (Bairagi 1980; Prahlad Rao 1980). Another important factor is sibling sequence. In North India, the second plus daughter has been shown to have a 70 percent greater risk of death before the age of five than the first daughter (Das Gupta 1987).

Social discrimination against female children, particularly in South Asia, has been documented and can have an impact on child nutrition (Chen *et al.* 1981; Carloni 1981). Conflicting results have emerged though. Studies in Nepal (Martorell *et al.* 1984), Sri Lanka (Perera 1983), and one in Bangladesh (Abdullah 1983) have found no gender differences in child growth retardation, while in two other studies in Bangladesh (Chen *et al.* 1981; Bairagi 1983) significantly more girls than boys under-five years old were found to be severely malnourished.

Finally, the politics of the control of food (Whitehead 1981) and health expenditure (Chen *et al.* 1981), and the quality of child care and feeding practices (De Chavez *et al.* 1974; Gopaldas 1983; Zeitlin 1985) may all have important nutritional consequences for children.

At the level of the individual, malnutrition has been shown to have a synergistic relationship with disease (Scrimshaw *et al.* 1968; Black *et al.* 1984; Tomkins and Watson 1988). Infections can lead to a loss of appetite (Mata et al 1977; Martorell *et al.* 1980), decreased efficiency of food and nutrient utilisation (Briscoe 1979), to increased energy requirements (Tomkins 1983), and to decreased rates of child growth (Rowland *et al.* 1977; Baumgartner and Pollit 1983). The relationship between diarrhoeal disease and physical growth in children has been shown in several studies to be particularly close (Levinson 1978; Chen *et al.* 1979; Prahlad Rao 1980; Martorell *et al.* 1984).

Malnutrition itself can lead to a greater susceptibility to infection due to the suppressive effect on the child's immune system (Tomkins 1986), and recent studies have shown that malnutrition is related more to the duration, severity and outcome of an illness, than to its incidence (Black *et al.* 1984; Tomkins 1986), although the latter may be associated with severe malnutrition. A number of studies are beginning to suggest nutritional benefits from improvements in water supply and/or sanitation, whether through diminished morbidity, savings in maternal time and energy, or improved food production, (Tomkins *et al.* 1978; Henry 1981; Tomkins 1983).

1.2 CONCEPTS AND DEFINITIONS

1.2.1 Nutritional Status

Anthropometric indicators, incorporating height and weight measurements, are most commonly used as proxies for 'nutritional status', an imprecise notion that represents the combined proximate outcome of the interaction between disease, access to care and food (Koenig and D'Souza 1986).

Nutritional status is an ambiguous concept. Firstly, it is used to refer to both the condition and the cause. Growth retardation can be a consequence of infection and disease and/or inadequate food intake, and so cannot be attributed solely to undernutrition. Secondly, the use of child nutritional status as a social indicator often rests on the assumption that the growth retardation of measured children says something meaningful about the rest of the population, unmeasured and adult.

In this study, nutritional status is proxied by growth retardation, as measured by anthropometry. The aetiology is not implied by the use of this term, and an attempt to classify households on the basis of the nutritional status of both adults and children will be made.

1.2.2 Malnutrition

Characteristic of much research in malnutrition is the assumption that malnutrition can be measured and interpreted. It is generally accepted that undernutrition or protein-energy malnutrition (PEM) is the most important nutritional problem in developing countries. Protein malnutrition is mainly a function of calorie malnutrition whereby protein sources are burned up to provide energy. Micronutrient deficiencies, possibly giving rise to detectable clinical signs, frequently occur in conjunction with PEM. In this study, 'malnutrition' refers to protein-energy malnutrition only.

The interpretation of anthropometric data often depends on reference norms, the value of which are now being debated both quantitatively (Lipton 1983) and conceptually (Payne 1985). Lipton claims that just as adult populations may live perfectly satisfactorily as smaller and lighter individuals than in the west, so children who are growing in trajectories parallel to western growth norms should not be classified as malnourished, unless their growth falters into the 'severe' category in which case physical and mental activity in the child may be impaired. Payne (1985) contrasts two 'theories' of how a person maintains the state of nutrition - the 'genetic potential' and 'adaptability' models. In the latter model, malnutrition is regarded as the result of the failure to maintain homeostatic control, and happens when an individual is forced beyond the limits of his/her adaptive range. In the former, malnutrition is seen as one of a range of sub-optimal states of nutrition.

Following Pacey and Payne (1985), malnutrition is defined in this study as: "a state in which physical function of an individual is impaired to the point where he or she no longer maintains adequate performance in such processes as growth, pregnancy, lactation or resisting and recovering from disease".

In children, evidence points to relatively small, or zero, functional losses accompanying a certain range of growth adjustments (Payne 1985). There is, however, more agreement about the implications of more severe degrees of growth retardation. In several South Asian studies, anthropometry has been shown to be a good predictor of mortality, at least for those individuals whose growth is badly affected.

In a study among Bangladeshi children, Chen *et al.* (1980) found there to be a threshold effect in which risk does not change according to anthropometric indices until a level (corresponding to the recognised cut-off for 'severe' malnutrition for three classification systems), is reached, at which mortality rates rise sharply. Bhan *et al.* (1986) in a study in Haryana, India, found diarrhoea-related mortality rates to be significantly higher among children with severe (weight-for-age) malnutrition as compared to other children.

In other studies, such as one in India by Keilmann and McCord (1978) and one in Papua New Guinea by Heywood (1986), there was a more linear relationship with steadily increasing mortality risk in relation to decreasing anthropometric indices. The relationship between anthropometry and subsequent risk of death was unimpressive in the Kasongo Project in Zaire (1986).

As regards the discriminatory power of anthropometric indicators, studies in Bangladesh by Chen *et al.* (1980), Bairagi *et al.* (1985) and Briend *et al.* (1986) all showed the weight-for-age index to be a particularly strong discriminator of mortality risk. In their review, Tomkins and Watson (1988) summarised these findings: "Overall there is a definite risk of mortality in relationship to growth. However, the strength of that relationship is likely to be relatively specific to the community and may be influenced by factors other than growth".

A single universal cut-off point at which mortality and morbidity increases cannot be established. However, studies carried out in South Asia tend to show that the 'state of severe malnutrition' as assessed against current international standards represents a meaningful state of physiological and social dysfunction with higher mortality risks than other classes of malnutrition, whether the relationship exhibits a 'threshold effect', or is more linear. As stated by Payne (1985): "It seems reasonable to accept any of the conventional systems of classifying 'severe' malnutrition for defining the break point at which anthropometry ceases to be a measure largely of the environment, and becomes an unequivocal index of personal risk to the individual"

In this study, special attention will be paid towards those children with 'severe' malnutrition. In Chapter 6, an in-depth investigation into the distinguishing socio-economic features of households containing a severely malnourished child, according to the Gomez weight-for-age classification, will be carried out. Children in the first or second degree categories of conventional classifications will here be referred to as being 'growth retarded'.

1.2.3 The Household

The concept of 'the household' implies a domestic unit with decision-making autonomy about production and consumption (Guyer 1986). White (1980) has pointed out that: "it is in fact their degree of autonomy of internal economic organisation relative to one another, rather than any particular uniformity in their organisation, which marks off 'household' units from each other". This autonomy, however, is not a manageable criterion for the isolation of household units in surveys, and it is thus necessary to compromise by selecting a more practicable criterion such as "cooking and eating together". For the purposes of this study, the functionalist definition of the household as a unit of consumption for subsistence, within which the reproduction of human labour or of the individual is assured, will be used. The use of the household level as a unit of data collection allows for analysis both at this level and, through aggregation and disaggregation, at community and individual levels.

It is not assumed by this that households act as homogeneous units. The study will recognise the possibility of divergence of interests between different family members and it will not be assumed that those who make the decisions regard the welfare of all household members as equally important. The South Asian household has been characterised as an arena for "co-operative conflict", where unequal intra-household material exchanges are culturally legitimated and co-exist with the common goal of increasing household entitlements (Sen 1987). In this study, therefore, the decision-making power of adult individuals within the household will also be examined.

1.3 TRIBAL ECONOMY AND SOCIETY

Most of the South Asian nutritional studies outlined above have been carried out in non-tribal villages. In order to fully understand the social and economic aspects of malnutrition and health in a tribal context, and the conceptual framework subsequently employed for the study, it is necessary at this stage to know something of tribal economy and society in India.

Corbridge (1988) has outlined three propositions that he believes together define a commonly held ideology of tribal economy and society. The first assumption of this ideology is that Indian tribals are typified by their geographical isolation and high levels of ethnic closure. Secondly, tribal communities lack an economic hierarchy and are egalitarian, and, thirdly, this supposed unimportance of economics is further underlined by the importance attached to cultural matters.

This ideology has been increasingly challenged within the last two decades. Corbridge himself (1986) has shown that none of these propositions appear to hold in the case of the tribals inhabiting the Jharkhand region of South Bihar. Beteille (1974) found a lack of correspondence befalling the claim that tribal societies are always 'isolated' and deprived of cultural contact with non-tribals. Asit Bandopadhyay, who was Land Reforms Commissioner in Bihar in 1977-79, has subsequently remarked (1979): "It is time to note that the many social and economic changes that have come about in tribal areas have created a class of tribal landholders and moneylenders who exploit small landholders of their own community".

With regard to religion, another common criterion for distinguishing tribal societies, Corbridge claims that in present-day India it is hard to find major tribal communities which exclusively practice animistic religions. According to Ghurye (1980), the 'animism' of tribal India has long been tinged with Hinduism, leading some authorities to maintain that India's 'animists' are best described as Backward Hindus. Beteille (1974) concluded his essay on Tribe and Peasantry by stating that in India, there really was no satisfactory way of defining a tribal society.

The study locality and characteristics of the tribal groups studied here are described in Chapter 2, while the levels of economic equality are examined in Chapter 3. In general, these criticisms of the propositions are felt by the investigator to hold for the tribals studied here, though in varying degrees.

1.4 CONCEPTUAL FRAMEWORK

The absence of a conceptual framework has often prevented nutrition studies with a socio-economic focus from organising the empirical information in terms of the central economic processes that characterise households. Frameworks often start with income and/or food availability, and fail to show the processes through which income is raised, or the mechanisms by which households become economically differentiated. Such an analysis needs to include the relations of production, circulation and reproduction.

The framework presented in Figure 1.1 is felt to be useful in accounting for variations in material conditions of tribal households and the nutritional and health outcomes of household reproduction.

It has been adapted from a framework used by Deere and de Janvry (1979) for the analysis of a peasant economy, in that it includes only those mechanisms of surplus appropriation (see 1.4.1) that exist in this increasingly commercialised tribal economy. Furthermore, cultural relations of production and reproduction (including gender) have been located in the framework, following Clark (1987).

An additional important dimension of this framework is time. Seasonality may affect child nutritional and health status through its effect on income, maternal time allocation and disease incidence. This effect is mediated by seasonality in waged and unwaged productive work, in wages and prices, in the division of family labour between productive and reproductive work, and in environmental conditions governing disease exposure.

Nine sets of variables were identified and located within the framework as a means of characterising household organisation. These are:

i) the stocks of means of production
ii) demographic characteristics and the division of productive labour
iii) home production process
iv) wage labour production process
v) disposal of the product
vi) distribution of income
vii) credit and debt
viii) effective demand - disposal of net income
ix) reproduction of the consumption unit (family labour)

FIGURE 1.1 : CONCEPTUAL FRAMEWORK OF PROCESSES OPERATING AT HOUSEHOLD LEVEL

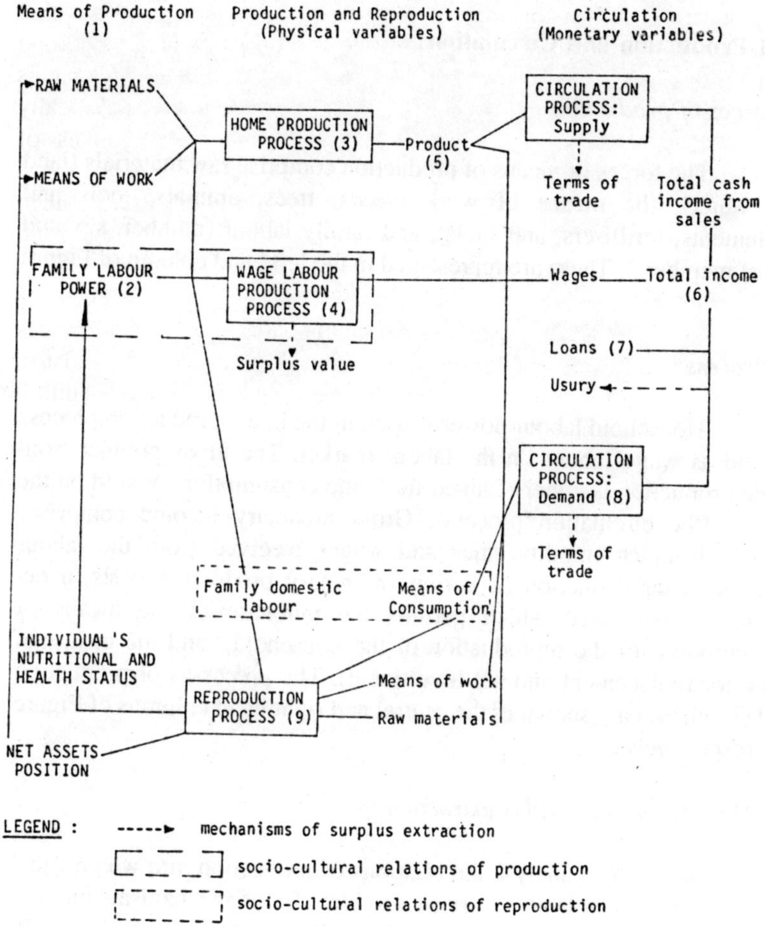

The processes of production, circulation and reproduction as described by these variables will be investigated in Chapter 3, while the nutritional and health outcomes will be dealt with in Chapter 4.

1.4.1 Production and Circulation

i) Forces of production

The forces or means of production comprise raw materials (land and water), the means of work (seeds, trees, animals, tools and implements, fertilisers, and fuels), and family labour (number, sex and age of members). These are represented in the left hand column of Figure 1.1.

ii) Process

Household labour power is used in the home production process or sold as wage labour on the labour market. The gross product from home production is either retained for home consumption, or sold on the market (the circulation process). Gross monetary income comprises income from commodity sales and wages received from the labour process. After deduction of various monetary production costs, a net income is generated which permits the purchase of the means of consumption for the reproduction of the household, (and the means of work for replacement and net investment). The processes of production and circulation are shown in the central and right hand columns of Figure 1.1 respectively.

iii) Mechanisms of surplus extraction

In order to analyse the relations of production into which tribal households enter, it is necessary first to identify the mechanisms through which extraction of surplus occurs. According to Athreya *et al.* (1987), surplus 'by definition' is what is available for luxury consumption or accumulation once simple reproduction of family (labour power) and farm (means of production) has been achieved. This surplus may be appropriated under production relations other than capitalist, either directly by the producers for savings or investment, or through secondary market relations of appropriation.

Deere and de Janvry identify seven mechanisms. Three operate via rents that result from private appropriation of land (rents in labour services, kind and cash), three operate via the markets (for labour, products and money), and one through the state (taxes). Of these, only the three that operate through the markets apply in this tribal context, and have been included in the framework. Rent exploitation does not occur and has been recognised as being much less prevalent than other forms of exploitation in dry areas of South India, such as this (Da Corta 1988). The mechanisms that apply operate:

(a) Via the labour process. Where the value of the product of labour is greater than the costs of replacement of the physical capital resources and the labour used in production, the profit thus generated represents surplus. Marginal farmers with insufficient land for household reproduction may be forced to sell their labour, as do all landless peasants. In so doing they may be further exploited indirectly as the male wage levels can fall below subsistence needs which are then partially met in the home production process. Women may be 'super-exploited', either through receiving lower wages than men for the same type of productive work, or through the unpaid labour carried out within the home. The latter raises the standard of living of household earners above that provided by the wage alone, and provides the services of care and socialisation of children who are the future labour force (Mackintosh 1981). This form of extraction will be investigated in the wage labour production process section.

(b) Via the terms of trade. Growing market relations are the driving force behind this type of surplus appropriation. Unfavourable price trends over time for commodities sold (including food) relative to the commodities purchased is the main mechanism here (Nadkarni 1980). This will be investigated in the sections on product disposal and effective demand.

(c) Via usury. Instability of agricultural production may force a dependence on local moneylenders who charge interest rates, higher than would be the case under conditions of competition (Bharadwaj 1974). If the moneylender is also a trader, the interlocking of money and food markets may further exploit indebted households by reducing their choice on other markets. This will be investigated in the credit and debt section.

iv) Social and cultural relations of production

The gender division of labour cannot be explained solely by the demands of a particular set of production relations. Rather, it may be understood in terms of the intersection of the relations of production with those of patriarchy, with the household as the mediating institution (Mackintosh 1981). Patriarchy is used here in its most general sense of the social dominance of the male. Once established, different areas of the sexual division of labour tend to reinforce one another e.g. the need to support and care for children may weaken women's bargaining position in the wage labour market.

The level of outcome of the production and circulation processes will determine the level of consumption possible to reproduce family labour.

1.4.2 Reproduction

i) Forces of reproduction

These comprise (a) the quantity and quality of family labour power, which is manifested by household size and composition and the nutritional, health and educational status of its members, (b) the means of consumption, or the combination of food available plus income for purchasing food and/or health care, and (c) the means of reproductive work i.e. water supply, housing, technologies for food preparation, cooking, sanitation and access to health care systems and technologies (e.g. medicines, contraceptives).

ii) Process

Human reproduction is a process whereby consumption is effected to restore or create the individual's capacity to work (1). The nutritional and health status of children (who are the labour force of the future) is one outcome, and can be considered as being a function of the quantity and allocation of income and time. Kumar (1983) terms the combination of income and time in this context, "household real income".

The availability of income at the household level determines food availability and thus represents the potential for adequate individual consumption. Time, on the other hand, needs to be allocated between such domestic tasks as cooking, repairing, post-harvest food processing and preparation, fuel and water collection as well as child care and feeding. Environmental conditions which govern disease exposure are also likely to be partially dependent on time spent cleaning the home. If a child becomes ill, further demands in terms of disease management and/or health service utilisation arise.

iii) Social and cultural relations of reproduction

These are located at the level of : (a) the household, in terms of how a family organises itself - the gender and generational division of domestic labour, decision-making power and control over resources, and, (b) the society, in terms of how households organise with respect to other households. This includes the system of control over resources transferred or reproduced socially via marriage and inheritance and the operational significance of religion and kinship, especially for female autonomy.

iv) Outcomes of the reproduction process

The framework illustrates how the nutritional and health status of children, is simultaneously an outcome and input into the processes of production and reproduction. Other material outcomes of less central concern to this study include net capital for investment, for working capital for tools and equipment.

1.5 CLASSIFICATION OF HOUSEHOLDS

In order to investigate socio-economic differentials in child nutritional well-being, it is necessary to classify the study households. Several methods were considered:

1.5.1 'Class'

'Class' has been operationalised by Patnaik (1979), following Marx, in terms of the household's position in the social organisation of the labour process, using a classificatory formula based on the relative levels of hired-in, hired-out and family productive labour (i.e. physical production variables, located in the central column of the framework). This was felt to be unsuitable for the following reasons: (a) it assumes homogeneity between the three types of labour, whereas, as pointed out by Athreya *et al.* (1987), it is widely recognised that the input of family labour by peasants on their own holdings follows another logic than their use of hired labour (2), (b) it does not take into account the effect of non-agricultural sources of income on labour use, nor labour exploitation in non-agricultural operations, (c) it does not incorporate relations of exploitation that operate through the processes of circulation, which are likely to be very important in this tribal context, (d) there is a lack of evidence of 'classes-in-themselves' (Byres 1981) i.e. there is a a general homogeneity with respect to structural relations of production and distribution. Sellers and purchasers of a commodity do not constitute two different classes, for the conflict of interest is not structural and comes into operation only under specific conditions, namely movement of prices. But landowners and tenants, industrial capitalists and wage labourers have conflicts of interest that are structurally based and hence more durable. These types of conflict, however, do not occur within these tribal villages, which may be regarded as residential and cultural, but not economic units. Economic processes act in the regional economy. For example, most of the moneylenders and traders related to the study households were based outside the study area, (e) There is also a lack of evidence of 'classes-for-themselves' (Byres 1981) within the villages, i.e. social groups, objectively defined by their structural relations, who perceive their common interests and thus exhibit a degree of class consciousness and behaviour.

1.5.2 'Entitlement'

Sen (1981) uses the word 'entitlement' to cover the set of resources and relationships determining command over food, and hence nutritional vulnerability. A household's entitlement has two dimensions - (a) ownership of the means of production, and (b) the potential provided by the exchange of any part of what is owned (a process termed 'exchange entitlement mapping' by Sen). In estimating food entitlement, the exchange potential of assets and income sources for food shows both the overall ability to command food and the relative importance of each type of entitlement.

Study households were classified according to their entitlement base (or available sources of income) in order to investigate the potential for differentiating types of household, and the results are outlined in

Appendix I.

In summary, although such a classification is more comprehensive methodologically than Patnaik's, inasmuch as it incorporates both labour and market exploitation, it is less specific empirically, because, in the study area, there was a marked homogeneity in the types of income sources available. Moreover, such a classification fails to take account of the quantity of income or assets possessed, which may well determine inter-household differences in, for example, the nature, motivation and extent of market involvement - factors likely to influence household food security and nutritional vulnerability.

1.5.3 Income

One argument, highlighted by Da Corta (1988), is that since no one indicator can incorporate all forms of exploitation, a simple economic categorisation with separate analytical treatment of these forms of exploitation would be superior. The use of household income as a classificatory variable is felt to be useful for other reasons: (a) it is an index of consumption which affects and is affected by nutrition and health. Hence it is appropriate for an analysis of reproduction and its nutritional and health outcomes, (b) it is a continuous variable which can be standardised with respect to the size and composition, and hence consumption requirements, of the household, (c) empirically, it was found to proxy for certain kinds of market involvement which influence food security, and differentiate households well with respect to other economic variables, particularly household wealth (see Chapter 3), (d) it is superior to landholding size, as it incorporates the effect of cropping patterns, irrigation, intensity of cultivation and non-farm activity which may differ between households, (e) it can be used cautiously to impute the value of unwaged labour, including time allocated to reproductive work within the household.

For these reasons, the variable 'total household income per consumption unit' was used as a basis for household classification. Total income was imputed as the aggregation of the value of the crops retained and allocated to debt repayment (valued at post-harvest prices) plus the value of crops sold (using prices received by the farmer), plus income from wage labour, asset sale and other sources (e.g. livestock, artisan work, salaried employment or gifts). Total income was standardised with respect to the consumption requirements of the household using

FIGURE 1.2 : DISTRIBUTION OF TOTAL HOUSEHOLD INCOME PER CU

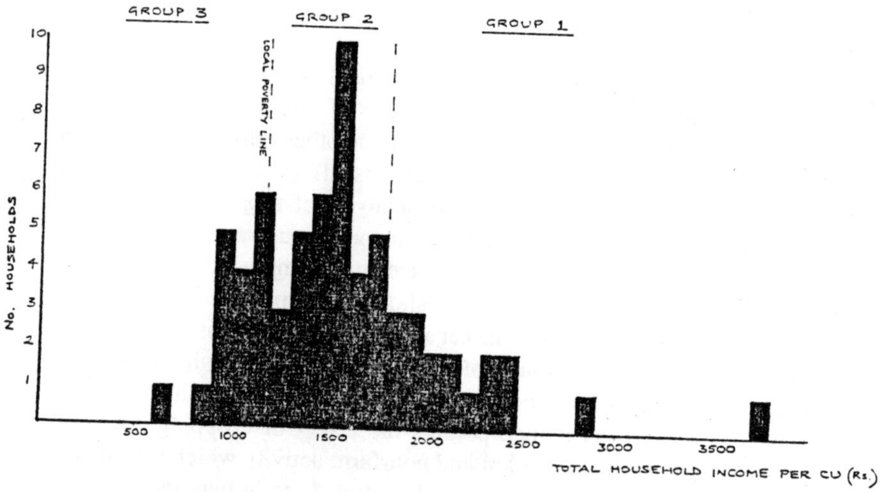

consumption units or adult equivalents as explained in Appendix II.

In order to differentiate households with respect to this variable, two consecutive steps were taken once the income distribution of study households had been plotted, as shown in Figure 1.2.

Firstly, the local poverty line (derived as described in Chapter 2 and Appendix III) was applied to the distribution, and those households below were defined as being the poorest 'Group 3'. One household whose income was fractionally above the line, but noticeably lower than the next household in the ranking, was included in this group giving a total of 17 households. The position of a household vis-a-vis the poverty line may be taken here as a proxy of the ability of a household to avoid reproductive crisis.

Secondly, the income distribution of those households remaining was examined to search for visible empirical clusterings of households. The distribution was skewed to the richer households, and a natural 'break-point' appeared to exist at the Rs. 1800 mark (approximately 1.5 times the local poverty line), delineating a middle 'Group 2', with 33 households, and the richest 'Group 1' with 17 households. The range of incomes in each group were of a similar magnitude, excepting one relatively very rich household in 'Group 1'. In this study, therefore, total household income per CU proxies for household socio-economic status.

1.6 STUDY HYPOTHESIS

The central hypothesis of this study emerges from the implications of the type of framework and household classification used. To recap : the notion of economic equality forms part of a commonly held ideology of tribal economy and society. Child nutritional and health status have been located as outcomes of a system of production and reproduction, and are thought to depend on the quantity and allocation of income and time. The mother's conflict between her need to combine productive with reproductive work may be intensified at certain times of the year, when female agricultural labour demand peaks. The effect of this conflict may be even more serious for the dependent child if seasonal peaks in labour demand and disease exposure coincide. The central hypothesis of this study is thus as follows :

> *'Within this tribal population, there is insufficient economic inequality for inter-household income differences to be related*

to child nutritional well-being. Rather, the latter is associated with seasonal peaks in maternal labour participation and child disease incidence'

In Chapter 2, the study area and population characteristics, criterion for household selection, types of data collected and methodology for analysis will be described. Chapter 3 comprises a socio-economic characterisation of the study households on the basis of those variables identified and located in the framework and a determination of the level of economic inequality within the study population. Chapter 4 describes the nutritional and health outcomes of the reproduction process - the type, severity and seasonality of child growth retardation and patterns of child morbidity, along with patterns of whole household anthropometry at one seasonal point.

The data on child nutritional and health status is related to the household socio-economic data and the hypothesis investigated in Chapter 5. The distinguishing features of households containing a severely malnourished child will be investigated in Chapter 6, and finally, the results and their practical implications are discussed and conclusions drawn in Chapter 7.

Notes

1. It is necessary here to distinguish several meanings of reproduction. The first has been called the reproduction of labour (Edholm *et al.* 1977) and involves the production of people - the bearing, care and socialisation of children and the maintenance of adults. Included within this is the narrower concept of human or biological reproduction (Bryceson 1980), the relations of which centre on the relations of marriage and kinship and construct the context for the bearing, care and socialisation of children. A further meaning, with which this study is not primarily concerned, is the concept of social reproduction - the process by which the main production relations are recreated and perpetuated.

2. Wage labour is employed until the marginal product is the wage, while family labour is used until the marginal product is zero.

2

CONTEXT AND METHOD

2.1 STUDY CONTEXT

2.1.1 Locality

The four small tribal villages in which the field research has been conducted are situated 50 km. north-east of the district capital, Warangal, in the government-reserved teak forest of the Telengana region; 200 km. from the Andhra Pradesh state capital, Hyderabad (see Figure 2.1). The nearest small market settlement is at Kothaguddem, 12 km. along a dirt road from the study villages. Kothaguddem is 16 km. from the nearest main market town in the plains, Narsampet, with only about half of the connecting road, surfaced.

2.1.2 Climate

In Telengana, the climate is semi-arid, markedly seasonal with a uni-modal rainfall, and would fall into classification E4 of Walsh's seasonality index (Walsh 1981). Summer lasts from March to mid-June, when temperatures regularly exceed 40 degrees Celsius and the relative humidity is 8-10%. The rainy season, from mid-June to September/October, begins with the arrival of the South-West monsoon which lowers the temperature by 5-10 degrees. The winter season, from October/November to January/February is generally rainless and cooler still, with maximum daytime temperatures ranging from the mid 20s to the low 30s Celsius. Monthly rainfall figures (in mm.) for the study year were obtained from the taluk headquarters and are presented in Table 3.3.

Agro-climatically, the forest area is one of relatively assured rainfall with medium-deep sandy loams. About 20 per cent of the total cropped area of the four villages is irrigated by the tank, which has, on average, 3-5 months per year irrigation capacity.

FIGURE 2.1 : STUDY LOCALITY

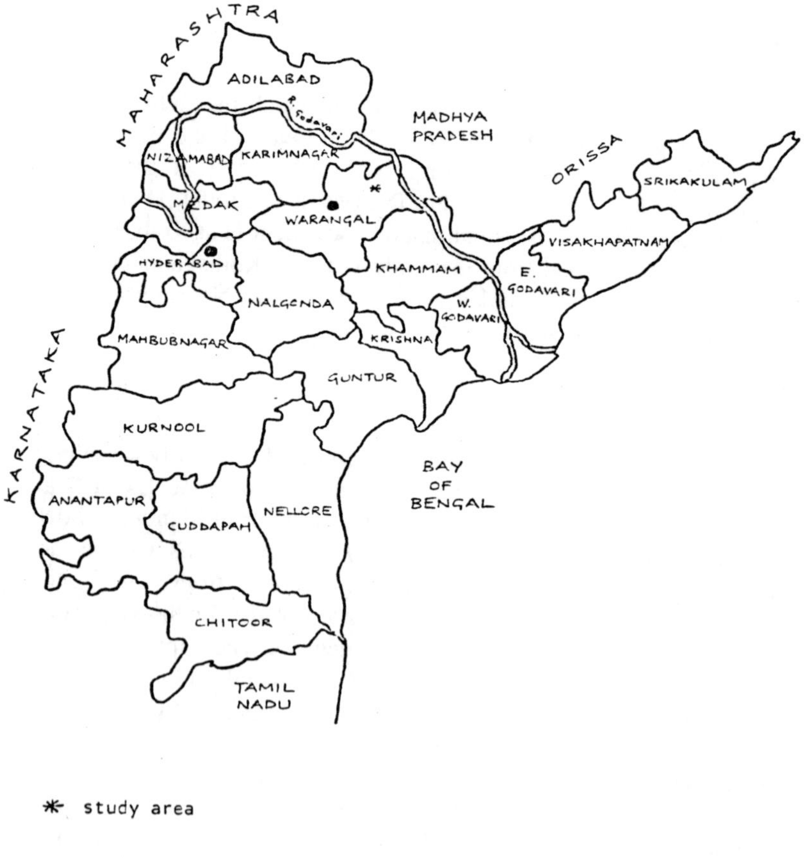

* study area

2.1.3 Tribal Groups

The tribes of Andhra Pradesh number approximately 1.5 million people and constitute nearly 4 per cent of the state's population (Von Furer-Haimendorf 1982). There are two main tribal groups in the study area. The Koyas are the largest tribe in Andhra Pradesh and the southern-most branch of the Gond tribe who inhabit the Warangal, Khammam, East and West Godavari districts (see Figure 2.1), predominantly the hilly regions. The Lambadis are a migrant group of North Indian descent, who have moved into the area in the last few decades, (many of whom were hired as construction workers to build the large dam at Nagarjunasagar). In 1977, Lambadis (or Banjaras) were included in the official government list of scheduled tribes thus legitimating land transfers between other tribals and themselves.

In the last two decades, as the population density has increased, the forest has become progressively depleted as more land is cleared for cultivation. According to Ramaiah (1981), the density of the tribal population in Narsampet taluk in 1981 (15 persons per sq. km.) was much higher than the average for the district (3 persons per sq. km.) and state (6 persons per sq. km.). In pursuit of the national policy on the problem of tribal land alienation, the Government of Andhra Pradesh has taken steps to protect and regulate tribal land rights. These are embodied in the Andhra Pradesh Scheduled Areas Land Transfer Regulations of 1959 and their 1978 Amendment. According to the latter, the Forest Department has the power to prevent land transfers from tribals to non-tribals, and to dispossess non-tribals illegally occupying tribals' land.

Non-tribals, however, have managed to move into the area from the plains (having often bribed officials), and set themselves up as traders and/or moneylenders. The low price of land, the availability of fuel and the tribal need for credit are the main incentives. Von Furer-Haimendorf (1982) refers to this influx and observes: "the ability of Koyas to retain their land stands in inverse relation to the accessibility of their villages".

Families are principally agrarian, with men and women working as cultivators on their own land or hiring themselves out as agricultural labourers. Very few households are landless, though landholdings are generally small in size, and predominantly rainfed. Forestry offers avenues of temporary employment in the non- agricultural summer months, when minor produce, such as bidi leaves, tamarind, mahua flowers, is gathered from the forest. Very few households had small-scale subsidiary occupations such as tailoring or basket-weaving.

2.1.4 Cultural Characteristics

The following characteristics describe the socio-cultural relations of reproduction at a societal level, as referred to in section 1.4.2.

Marriage

Both tribal groups are basically monogamous, while tribal endogamy is absolute. Many marriages involve close kin in other villages and are parentally arranged. Wives remove to the husband's house which is often his parental home. Most girls are married before the age of sixteen. Basic marriage expenses are met by the bride's parents and a gift e.g. a watch, cycle or radio, may be presented to the groom's father. Dowry is becoming increasingly widespread and the amounts of dowry stipulated at marriage are increasing as the tribals are becoming more exposed to external Hindu customs.

Inheritance of farmland

The transmission of farmland to sons, either on the death of the father or when the son starts cultivating separately, is far more common than selling, for both tribal groups. Property is divided equally among the male members. If the husband dies, the wife also gets one share along with her sons. Laws that decree that daughters as well as sons should inherit a share of their father's property are largely ignored.

Religion

The tribals have traditionally worshipped several forest goddesses e.g. Mamili and Mutyalamma; each one of whom is linked to some aspect of agriculture, health or fertility. For example, in some Koya villages a goat may be sacrificed to Mamili to ensure good crop yields. Mutyalamma is supposed to preside over smallpox and cholera. In each village, there is a female 'messenger' through whom the goddess may be 'reached'. There is widespread belief that the contracting of a disease e.g. dysentery, is due to neglect of a particular goddess.

Over the last two decades, however, a process of Hinduization has been occurring in the forest, although several of the ritual trappings of animism still exist. Goat sacrifices only occur in a few particularly remote villages and the festivals of Dussera, Deepavalli and Sankranti are widely celebrated amongst the tribals of this area. Wealthier households have been known to make pilgrimages to Hindu temples in Tirupati, south Andhra.

2.1.5 Village Characteristics

Two of the study villages are Koya - Musmi and Bottevenniguddem - while two are Lambadi - Musmi Thanda and Ravenniguddem (although in the latter village, there are three Koya households). No non-tribal households exist in the study villages, though there are several in less remote villages, nearer Kothaguddem. The villages are all clustered around a lake or tank which is a common source of irrigation for several households. The entire cluster of villages is locally referred to as Musmi Gumpu (group).

Houses are randomly grouped and made of bamboo trellis walls, plastered over with mud, with mud floors and thatched roofs. Sanitation levels are poor. The universal practice is to defaecate in the forest beyond the tree line after dawn, in locally recognised male and female areas. There is no electricity, though this is scheduled to be introduced by 1990. Water is drawn from public wells. A borewell was sunk in each village in 1984, though a year later, they had all either broken or dried up, and had not been repaired or replaced.

Formal education facilities are inaccessible. The nearest government-sponsored day school is 10 km. away in Vellubelle. The few children from the study villages that attend, do so usually only in the summer months.

2.1.6 Health Care

Allopathic treatment is virtually non-existent in the study area. The nearest Primary Health Care centre is 25 km. away in Gudur, which is even more inaccessible than Narsampet, there being just two buses per day from Kothaguddem. Those that do make the trip often find the doctor absent. There are several expensive private clinics in Narsampet. Alternatives include the local Registered Medical Practitioner (RMP), who practises a combination of homeopathy and allopathy part-time, and local healers who may perform mantras and dispense 'chettlu mandullu' (literally 'tree medicine').

2.1.7 Dietary Patterns

Major subsistence crops grown in the villages are paddy, sorghum (jowar) and maize. Small quantities of pulses, particularly pigeon pea (redgram) are occasionally planted. Land that can be tank-irrigated will be set aside for paddy cultivation while maize and jowar are usually rainfed crops on dry land.

The most common food preparation, eaten with rice, particularly in the summer, is 'pulsu' (tamarind extract mixed with jaggery and ground sesame seeds) or 'pachapulsu' (a chutney of green chillies). Small quantities of pulses, particularly redgram, may also be mixed as a thin soup into the rice. The consumption of vegetables e.g. onions, eggplant, gourds, beans, tomatoes and greens, is largely determined by availability and income; they are consumed predominantly in the rainy season. Wild foods from the forest e.g. custard apples, mahua fruits, are also consumed, particularly in late summer.

Meat, such as chicken, goat or occasionally beef, is eaten maybe once every 1-2 weeks by richer families and by most households during festivals or weddings. Fish from the tanks or run-off channels ('wagoos'), are caught and eaten in mid-rains.

Milk is rarely consumed. Alcohol, particularly 'saara' - a spirit distilled from the flowers of the mahua tree - is drunk habitually by the great majority of men. There are generally no foods specifically restricted to men or women. The diets of both tribal groups are similar, except for the consumption by Lambadis alone of sorghum.

Infants are generally breast fed exclusively up to the age of 6-8 months, or maybe older, after which time the child is gradually weaned on to softened rice, maize gruels, or, more often, directly on to the adult diet. A mother may often decide to postpone weaning until the child appears strong enough to cope with solid food. Hence, a vicious circle may come into play, whereby a malnourished child is fed solely on breast milk for longer, thus perpetuating his/her malnutrition as the calorific adequacy of the breast milk intake decreases progressively. Weaning may also be delayed if the child is anorexic; a condition possibly brought on by chronic illness.

Breast feeding is generally only terminated when the mother becomes pregnant again. Otherwise, it may even continue until the child is four years old. Most mothers believe that lactation is established only two or three days after delivery, so the infant is usually put to the breast on the third day. During the first twenty- four hours, the majority of the new-borns receive water sweetened with either sugar or jaggery.

2.2 DATA AND METHOD

In this section, the types and uses of data collected and the methodology of analysis are described in two sub-sections - 'production and reproduction' and 'nutritional and health outcomes', following a description of the study household selection procedure. The fieldwork was carried out entirely by the investigator between February 1985 and February 1986, his having spent one year prior to the study associated with a rural development project in another tribal village, 5 km. from the study area. Data analysis was carried out in four stages : coding, computer data-entry, editing, followed by descriptive and inferential statistical analysis. Anthropometric transformations were analysed with socio-economic variables using the SPSSx statistical package (SPSS Inc. 1983).

2.2.1 Selection of the Study Households

TABLE 2.1 : VILLAGE DISTRIBUTION OF THE STUDY COMMUNITY

Village	Population	Total Households	Study Households	Under-fives
Musmi	126	25	15	24
Bott'guddem	107	21	13	20
Musmi Thanda	128	23	14	24
Ravenniguddem	212	39	25	44
Total :	573	108	67	112

A demographic census was carried out in February 1985 in the four villages, when data were collected on household size and the age and sex of its members. Households were subsequently selected on the basis of a single criterion : the presence in the household of at least one child under the age of five years. 67 households were thus selected, and their distribution between villages is shown in Table 2.1

2.2.2 Production and Reproduction

The data collected to describe these two processes are sub-divided here into the sets of variables located in the framework (see Figure 1.1).

i) Means of production

The following types of data were collected from each household at the beginning of the study in March 1985 and again in February 1986 (to assess the degree of asset sale or purchase within the study period):

- Landholding type, cultivated acreage and major crops grown (raw materials).
- Ownership of productive assets (means of work), such as livestock (bullocks, cows, goats, chickens), ploughs, wells, carts etc.
- Ownership of non-productive consumer durables, such as radios, cycles, watches.

These assets were valued at average local prices prevailing at the time, and having ascertained the value of wet and dry land from the village sarpanch, a composite figure for total asset value was computed for each household.

ii) Demographic characteristics and the division of productive labour

These were determined using the data on household size and composition, collected in the initial demographic census. The gender division of productive labour was revealed through the anthropological technique of participant observation, and during the time allocation studies described below.

iii) Home production process

Labour participation. The number of days spent on on-farm work or minor forest produce gathering by each adult was estimated by fortnightly recall. Co-operative (or exchange) labour arrangements existed, whereby family labour was reciprocally exchanged between different households. The amount of this type of labour was small as compared to on-farm or wage labour. As the exchange uses family labour, it is treated here as being equivalent to family or on-farm labour, as suggested by Athreya *et al.* (1987).

Crop production. Crop yields were recorded at the time of harvest, by recall of the male household head.

iv) Wage labour production process

Labour participation. The number of days spent by each adult on different types of wage labour was estimated by fortnightly recall. Types of labour included agricultural, migrant work, salaried employment, contractual forest produce gathering, artisanship and local non-agricultural labour.

Wages and individual incomes. The wages received were recorded at the same time, enabling a computation of individuals' income earned from each source. Gender differences in wage rates were examined to reveal the existence, if any, of super-exploitation of women over men in the labour market.

Livestock income. Income received through the hiring out of livestock was recorded.

v) Disposal of the produce

As the decisions for disposal of produce were generally made soon after the harvest, the monetary values of the quantities sold, retained for home consumption or allocated to debt repayment were recorded. The prices received for produce sold were recorded, while the prevailing crop market values were used to impute the value of crops not sold. This data reveals the extent of participation in the crop market and enabies an investigation into whether poorer households are discriminated against with respect to the local terms of trade.

vi) Distribution of income

Poverty. The prevalence and intensity of poverty in the study population was examined by evaluating income distributions against national and local poverty lines.

In 1981, the Government of India released revised figures for the 'official' national Indian poverty line in rural areas: Rs. 65 per capita per month. This was derived from Dandekar and Rath's calorie poverty line of Rs. 15 per capita per month at 1960-61 prices (1971), and is defined in the Sixth Five Year Plan as being the mid point of the monthly expenditure class having a daily per capita calorie intake of 2,400 kilocalories. In order to adjust for inflation between 1960 and 1985, Dandekar and Rath's line was multiplied by a factor of six, to give a calorie poverty line at 1985 prices of Rs. 90 per capita per month or Rs. 1080 per capita per annum (1).

The percentage of household income allocable to food expenditure has been taken here to be 70%, as originally suggested by Patnaik (1976). This is a generous allowance - several reports have suggested 80% should be used. However, here we are comparing the poverty line to gross rather than net income, hence underestimating the extent of actual poverty. The median percentage of gross household income allocated to food expenditure was, in fact, 72 percent.

In order to avoid the controversy surrounding the relevance of an adjusted national norm, a local food poverty line was constructed. This was based on a weighted basket of the aggregation of production plus purchases minus sales of the most commonly consumed foods in the three main food categories i.e. rice, redgram and oil. Appendix III shows calculation of the daily cost, at 1985 prices, of sufficient calories of such a food basket, for one adult equivalent or consumption unit.

Ultra poverty. An attempt to avoid problems of poverty lines' being defined with respect to the investigator's valuation of what should be regarded as being unacceptable, has been made by Lipton (1983). He introduced 'objective' behavioural criteria into the definition of a poverty line, by observing how the poor express their own valuations through their food expenditure patterns.

Lipton takes 20% as being the irreducible proportion of income spent by the poorest in a wide range of countries on non-food essentials. Given the tendency of food requirement figures to over- estimate real food needs, especially in relation to people living in warm climates,

Lipton suggests that it might be more realistic to work with 80% of the FAO/WHO weight-adjusted dietary energy requirements (FAO/WHO 1973), this leads to a 'double 80' rule, according to which people are judged to be 'ultra poor' if 80% of their income is insufficient to purchase 80% of these FAO/WHO energy requirements.

According to Lipton, for most low income countries, 10-20% households fall into these ultra-poor groups, and their members, especially children, are at quite substantial risk of becoming severely undernourished if the ultra-poverty is long sustained. Lipton also claims the 'ultra poor' are distinguishable by the perverse nature of their income/expenditure relationships. They are said to flout the laws of food behaviour, described in sub-section (8).

Inequality. Inequality and poverty are not unrelated, though neither concept subsumes the other. To determine whether this tribal society is egalitarian , two methods were used: i) Examination of the shares of the aggregate income and asset value owned by the top 20% as compared to the bottom 20% of households ranked in descending order according to these two variables. These are shorthand indicators of income and asset distribution. ii) Calculation of an index of inequality, the Gini or Concentration Coefficient, and its representation by a Lorenz curve (see Appendix IV).

Results were compared with those from other studies of agrarian inequality in tribal and non-tribal villages in South India.

vii) Credit and debt

The amount, source, interest rate and repayment conditions of all loans taken were recorded as and when they were contracted. This revealed the dependence of households on institutional or private sources and the existence, if any, of discrimination against the poorest borrowers in the operation of the money market.

viii) Effective demand - disposal of net income

Expenditure data were collected at three mid-seasonal points corresponding to mid-summer (April), mid-rains (August) and mid-winter (December), and sub-divided into the following categories: staple foods (predominantly rice), meat, pulses, vegetables, spices and oil, liquor and tobacco, health (including cost of treatment, medicines and transport).

Staple foods, spices, cooking oil and tobacco were generally bought monthly in bulk from the nearest fair-price shop in Kothaguddem, while weekly purchases were made of other foods from local shops or travelling traders. Liquor was often bought on a daily basis. For these reasons, the data were collected by a detailed weekly recall method in the middle of the months specified above, with care being taken to elicit the bulk expenditure at the fair- price shop and the interval between visits to it. Recalls were taken from the male household head, usually in the evening in the presence of his wife. The data were aggregated to give a monthly figure for each of the three seasons. The prices paid for foodstuffs were elicited to determine whether the retail food market discriminated against poorer households with respect to price.

Compliance with two of the three laws of food behaviour was also investigated (2). These laws are as follows:

> *Engel's Law.* As income rises, the proportion of income spent on food declines.
> *Law of Starchy Staples.* As income rises, inferior staples are substituted by higher quality and/or higher priced staples.

The food behaviour exhibited by those households defined as being 'ultra poor' was examined to assess aspects of deviance from these laws.

ix) Reproduction of the consumption unit

Data was collected on household energy consumption and parental time allocation to characterise the reproduction process, while data on parental decision-making involvement was collected to throw some light on the gender relations of household reproduction.

Household energy consumption. The amounts of staple foods consumed daily by each household at three seasonal points (March, July and December) were estimated by 24 hour recall of the mother, with the aid of a locally used grain measure, the 'chumbu'. The mother was asked to measure out, into a household seive, using a 'chumbu', the quantity of dry rice she intended to cook that day, and to state how long this would feed the family. The number of 'chumbus' was recorded and later converted into calories using the Food Composition Tables (NIN 1984). Where rice had been kept overnight for consumption, its equivalent in dry rice was also estimated.

The measurement of individual food intake was not undertaken for several reasons. Firstly, there are problems of reliability where trade-offs between precision, on the one hand and invasiveness, time and cost on the other, are necessary. Secondly, it was not possible to estimate the caloric contribution of breast milk intake, nor of 'snacking', and, thirdly, recognition of the possibility of adaptations in metabolism and in activity to fluctuations in food intake make them difficult to interpret, either per se, or in relation to 'problematical' concepts of requirements (Pacey and Payne 1985).

Time allocation. The time allocation of the mother and the father (3) in a sub- sample of 24 households, at three mid-seasonal points, was recorded. The daily time spent on productive and reproductive activities, especially child care, was thus estimated and the gender division of labour illustrated.

These studies were carried out between the 27th-30th. of March, July and November. One village was studied per day from dawn until dusk. A stratified random sub-sample of the study households was chosen in the following way:

i) only households containing a child under 24 months of age were initially considered. As the time allocated to child care was of prime importance to the central hypothesis, it was felt necessary to target those households with children who were particularly dependent on the mother.

ii) these households were then sub-divided into three groups on the basis of their composite landholding size - a variable that roughly proxies for the classificatory variable, income (which had not been determined at the beginning of the study) (4). The three groups were as follows : under 2 acres; 2-4 acres; over 4 acres.

iii) two households were chosen at random from each of these three groups in each of the four villages, giving a total of 24 households.

The technique of 'random instants' observation developed by White (1984) was used. This was a pragmatic compromise between the continuous observation and recall methods in terms of reliability, invasiveness and feasibility. Each sample household was visited every 20 minutes and the activities of the adults at the precise moment of the visit recorded. Owing to the proximity of the villagers' land to their homes, it was possible to obtain at least 30 'instants' per person during each day.

The validity of the results will be limited by the sample size and the limited periods of observation. Nevertheless, this technique was felt to provide a rough composite picture of time allocation and the gender division of labour in the study community. The activities recorded for each respondent were classified into seven categories: communal, non-agricultural/wage labour, non-agricultural/own labour, agricultural/wage labour, own agriculture, child care, other domestic.

The 'other domestic' category includes socially reproductive activities such as post-harvest food processing and preparation, washing clothes and utensils, collecting water and fuel, house cleaning and repairing clothes. Many activities were carried out simultaneously, e.g. child care and cooking. In these situations, the activity that was given the most attention (as observed by the researcher) determined its classification. For example, where a mother was caring for her child while rice was cooking, this was classified as 'child care'. Where she was pounding rice, with the child nearby, this was classified as 'other domestic' work.

Activities carried out during the researcher's meal breaks were recalled by the respondent directly afterwards. Leisure time, including sleep, is a residual, which was not directly quantified.

Decision-making. As a means of investigating aspects of the socio-cultural relations of reproduction that determine how a household organises itself internally, the relative participation of men and women in decisions relating to expenditure on production, consumption and health, was examined. An essentially 'qualitative' case-study approach to data collection was used which also allowed for quantitative analysis and presentation of results.

Over the study period, field notes were collected for each household in the course of the regular interviews on actual decisions made and by whom. In this way responses were thought to reflect the actual spheres of influence of individual husbands and wives, rather than socially acceptable norms about who ought to control decisions. Interviews therefore were necessarily open-ended and geared to, wherever possible, eliciting concrete cases of decisions recently made.

A cumulative picture of the pattern of decision-making in each household was thus constructed. The raw data were later converted into summary form, whereby each couple was placed along a scale in each area of decision-making, with decisions made by 'wife alone' and 'husband alone' at each extreme and an intermediate category of 'joint decision'. It is not, however, realistic to suppose the results were free from the preconceptions and values of either the respondents or the researcher. Examples of the type of decisions made in the 'food' category include the amount and proportion of household income spent on food and the quantity and types of food purchased.

2.2.3 Nutritional and Health Outcomes

In order to investigate the prevalence, severity and seasonality of child growth retardation, anthropometric data was collected monthly for under-five year old children. Intra-household patterns of adult and child anthropometry at one seasonal point were also examined. Finally, the nature, incidence and seasonality of disease among under-fives were investigated using morbidity recall data collected regularly from the child's mother.

Anthropometry

Under-five year old children. The weight and height of each child under five years old were monitored monthly. All measurements were taken at the beginning of each month according to standardised methodologies (Jelliffe 1966).

Salter 0-25 kg. scales were used to measure the child's weight to the nearest 100g. These were calibrated daily and the standardisation re-checked at the completion of field work. All subjects wore very light clothing and no footwear during the weighings. Standing heights were measured to the nearest 1 mm. using a locally-constructed measuring board. For infants, recumbent length was measured using a wooden 'length board'. Repeatability trials for weight and height measurement were carried out and the extent of intra-observer error was found to be negligible.

The age of the child was determined through discussion with the mother with the aid of a local events calendar (similar to the activity calendar shown in Table 3.3.).

Both Western and Indian standards were used to analyse the anthropometric data of under-fives. The Indian standards used were those supplied by the National Institute of Nutrition (Ryan *et al.* 1984). These data were provided by Hyderabadi children of diverse, but predominantly

Telegu, backgrounds who were for the most part, from the middle socio-economic class, or above. The Western standards used were those published by WHO (WHO 1983). These calculations use data from the National Center for Health Statistics (NCHS) as standards (NCHS 1977).

Three anthropometric measures were used as proxy indicators of nutritional status, based on the NCHS standards. The abbreviations subsequently used are in parentheses:

> Weight-for-age (WA) - generally accepted as a measure of overall nutritional status, being a composite indicator of both long-term and current growth retardation.
> Height-for-age (HA) - generally accepted as a measure of stunting and indicating long-term or 'chronic' growth retardation.
> Weight-for-height (WH) - generally accepted as a measure of wasting and indicating recent or 'acute' growth retardation.

In addition, the weight velocity of study children was determined by calculating the mean weight gains for each month. A reduction in weight velocity is recognised as a particularly sensitive index of growth failure (Nabarro 1984).

In order to investigate the effects of seasonality and household socio-economic status on the nutritional status of children, the Z- score computation of the anthropometric data was adopted. Mean Z- scores of anthropometric indices for children in each age-sex category were plotted for each month.

The seasonal variations in the proportions of children suffering wasting and stunting, according to the Waterlow (1972) classification, were also investigated using Z-scores. The monthly measurements for weight and height, expressed simply as greater or less than 2 standard deviations (SD) below the NCHS median weight- for-height and height-for-age, (i.e. with a Z-score of less than - 2.00), were cross-tabulated to determine the monthly prevalences of 'wasting', 'stunting' and 'wasting and stunting combined'. Children whose weight was more than 2 SD below the reference median weight- for-height were labelled as 'wasted', while those whose height was more than 2 SD below the reference median height-for-age were defined as 'stunted'. Children suffering neither wasting nor stunting were considered 'normal'. Using these definitions, the sex-specific prevalences of wasting and stunting were compared.

The application of Z-scores represents one approach to the setting up of cut-off points. These have recently been suggested for adoption by WHO (1983). In most of the studies reviewed earlier, anthropometric indicators of populations were expressed as mean Z-scores or mean percentages of the reference. Findings by Hernandez *et al.* (1974) have suggested that anthropometry should be expressed both ways. Indian studies in the past have tended to use the cut-off points, based on the percentage of the median of the reference population, suggested by Gomez *et al.* (1955) for weight-for-age and Waterlow *et al.* (1972) for height-for-age and weight-for height. These are :

> Weight-for-age : more than 90% normal; 75-90% first degree; 60-74%, second degree; less than 60%, severely underweight.
> Height-for-age : more than 95%, normal; 90-95%, first degree; 85-89%, second degree; less than 85%, severe stunting.
> Weight-for-height : more than 90%, normal; 80-89%, first degree; 70- 79%, second degree; less than 70%, severe wasting.

In order to compare the results of this study with previous rural India-based nutritional studies, the annual mean proportions of children falling into these categories were determined. Furthermore, in order to investigate the socio-economic features of households containing the most malnourished children in the study population, the Gomez weight-for-age cut-off for 'severe' malnutrition was used, for the reasons stated in section 1.2.2.

For subsequent analyses, the anthropometric data were classified into age-sex groups. Three age groups were used that corresponded with WHO recommendations for study samples of this magnitude (Waterlow *et al.* 1977): i) less than 12 months, ii) 12 to 23 months, and iii) 24 to 60 months.

The age of the child at the beginning of the study period (i.e. March 1985) was used in classification. This age classification was also locally relevant, in that it corresponded roughly to the three stages of child feeding i.e. breast feeding, weaning period, adult diet.

Whole household anthropometry. By extending the unit of measurement from the individual to the household, patterns of intra-household anthropometry which characterise different problems and causes may be distinguished and problem families in which malnutrition and disease tend to cluster, identified (Dugdale 1985). Families with very low food entitlement may be identified, without having to rely on measurements made on a single individual (who may be undersized, for reasons other than food shortage), and whole household anthropometry may also provide some measure of intra-household distribution which does not entail making assumptions about relative food requirements of individual members. Such an approach has been advanced as being of potential use in targeting household nutrition interventions more accurately and efficiently.

Weight and height measurements for each family were taken in the first week of August 1985, in the middle of the rainy season, directly after a period of high adult work load (particularly for women), and at a time when childrens' nutritional status was seen to generally be at a particularly low level. Weights of older children and adults were measured with bathroom scales.

A weight-for-height indicator was used, it being the best indicator of present nutritional status and applicable to all age groups. For under thirteen year olds, a cut-off of 90% NCHS standard weight-for-height (WH) was employed (it being widely accepted as the lower limit of 'normal' (Waterlow 1972)). For adolescents, as the standard measurements of WH vary widely with age due to the 'growth spurt' occurring in this age group, an age-independent WH index for adolescents, devised by Dugdale (1987) was used.

For adults, body mass index (BMI or weight/ (height*height)) was used, as suggested by Dugdale (1985) and Payne (1985). There is no BMI cut-off which is generally accepted as marking the dividing line between an acceptable state of health and malnutrition. Ferro-Luzzi *et al.* (1988) have carried out a review of studies that have tried to use BMI as an indicator of undernutrition in adults. They state that "from an operational point of view, there may be an advantage in having a graded classification, of the kind traditionally used for the assessment of PEM in children".

They go on to suggest three cut-off points on the basis of the evidence of the studies reviewed: BMI values of 20, 18.5 and 17. A BMI of 20 represents the upper limit for a diagnosis of undernutrition. A BMI of 17 or below is taken as too low and as constituting a risk to health. Between 17 and 20, however, the picture is not nearly so clearcut, so the mid-point of 18.5 is arbitrarily chosen. The cut-off of 18.5 was chosen as the cut-off point for the household anthropometric profiles, with a separate breakdown of the adult BMI values into categories defined by all three cut-offs.

For the purpose of this classification, only BMIs of the childrens' parents were included. This was obviously a simplification (although 80% of households were nuclear), which also served to demonstrate the potential limitations of classification systems for such data, where trade-offs between the number of patterns delineated and their practical utility may need to be made. As with other types of data in this study, attention has been focused on the parents.

Morbidity

Morbidity data for each under-five child were collected twice per month by maternal recall. The disease categories were derived according to local perceptions. (5)

The investigator felt that such morbidity data was unlikely to be of sufficient reliability for multiple disease episodes within each month to be differentiated. Frequency of diarrhoeal episodes, for example, is an elusive concept, especially in circumstances where diarrhoea tends to be a chronic, continuing phenomenon. Rowland *et al.* (1977) estimate that the average rural Gambian infant spends 20.4% of the rainy season with diarrhoea. In such circumstances, the boundary between one episode and the next becomes blurred. Hence, the monthly incidence risk (Kirkwood 1988) here refers to the probability (expressed as a percentage) that a child, initially free from a disease, starts at least one disease episode within the month. The data were disaggregated by sex, age, income group and season to provide a morbidity profile of the study children.

Parental perceptions of seasonal family vulnerability to ill-health and the relationship between the seasonality of health expenditure and child morbidity were also investigated.

Notes

1. The change of gold price in the villages was used as an index of inflation, as suggested by Jodha (1983). The logic in this is that one Tola (10g.) of gold fetched roughly the same quantity of rice in 1985 as it did in 1960, but gold price per Tola has increased by about six times since then.

2. Owing to the lack of data on total household cash expenditure, Bennet's Law could not be investigated. This law states that, as income rises, the proportion of total expenditure allocated to cereals declines.

3. For reasons of inter-household standardisation and practical feasibility, the time allocation studies were confined to the parents.

4. The correlation between composite landholding size and household income was found to be high ($r = 0.73$; $P<0.01$) (see section 3.1.1).

5. As suggested by Dubos (1979) : "Health and disease cannot be defined merely in terms of anatomical, physiological or mental attributes. The real measure is the ability of the individual to function in a manner acceptable to himself and to the group of which he is part".

3

HOUSEHOLD PRODUCTION AND REPRODUCTION

In this chapter, a socio-economic characterisation of the study households will be developed and the range of material conditions and mechanisms of surplus appropriation described. The analysis of production, circulation and reproduction will be disaggregated by income group, and by season and gender where the latter are relevant. Tribal differences in various socio-economic factors will be highlighted where they are statistically significant, at the 5% level.

The sets of key variables identified and located in the framework will be used to structure the analysis. One-way analysis of variance will be employed to detect significant differences ($P<0.05$) between income-group means for various factors (1), while a Scheffe test will enable the individual groups that are significantly different to be pinpointed.

Where distributions are severely non-normal and/or standard deviations of the three groups are very different, the one-way analysis of variance test is contraindicated (Kirkwood 1988). In these situations, logarithmic transformations of the data will be performed to remove skewness of distribution or equalize the standard deviations, prior to the test. In the tables in this chapter, data for asterisked (*) variables has been 'logged', and the significance values refer to the results of the test carried out on this 'logged' data, although the original means and standard deviations are shown.

Linear trends in association between various factors and the classificatory variable - total household income per CU - will be investigated using correlation analysis. Seasonality is explored by dividing the year into three main locally-recognised seasons, which are:
- *summer*: hot, dry, post-harvest, little farm activity (March to May).
- *rains*: monsoon, pre-harvest, high farm activity (June to September).
- *winter*: cool, dry, harvest, moderate farm activity (October to February).

For the sake of clarity, the abbreviations G1, G2 and G3 will be used to refer to the three income-groups; G1 being the richest and G3, the poorest.

3.1 MEANS OF PRODUCTION

3.1.1 Land

Most families 'owned' their land; there were no landlords leasing out large tracts, and virtually no sharecropping. It was difficult, however, to ascertain whether a family had legal land rights ('pattas'), for each plot it farmed. Clearing of forest land for cultivation without prior application for pattas was not uncommon. Of the 67 study households, 3 were landless, 19 cultivated less than 2 acres, 35, between 2 and 4 acres, and 10, more than 4 acres.

Paddy was, by far, the most important crop. The two other main subsidiary crops were maize and sorghum. All households with land grew paddy, whilst 54% and 61% households grew maize and sorghum respectively. There were highly significant income-group differences in the cultivated acreages of paddy and maize (but not sorghum) as shown in Table 3.1. A composite indicator of the total operational landholding size per CU (standardised according to average village yield values of the three main crops) also showed a highly significant income-group difference, and correlated very significantly ($r=0.73; P<0.01$) with total household income per CU. This indicates the importance of land as a source of income.

3.1.2 Total Assets

Total asset value per CU, the bulk of which was land value, showed highly significant income-group differences, with the Group 1 mean being three times that of Group 3. Socio-economic differences in the ownership of assets other than land were not great. An 'average' household might have owned : 2 bullocks, 3 cows, 2 goats, 4 chickens and 1 plough. Only 20% households owned a bullock cart; 13%, a well; 27%, a radio; 15%, a cycle and 15%, a watch. There was a very significant positive association ($r=0.82; P<0.01$) between total asset value per CU and total household income per CU, indicating the predominance of owned assets as sources of income.

3.2 DEMOGRAPHIC CHARACTERISTICS AND THE DIVISION OF PRODUCTIVE LABOUR

3.2.1 Household Type

The types of study households falling into four categories, commonly recognised by demographers, are described below. Percentages refer to the proportion of households in each category:

Nuclear (one couple plus any children): 80.6%
Supplemented nuclear (nuclear plus a relative): 9.0%
Lineal joint (more than one couple of two generations): 9.0%
Collateral joint (more than one couple of the same generation): 1.4%

3.2.2 Household Size

The mean study household size was 5.5 members, ranging from 3 to 9 members. Poorer households had more 'dependent CUs' (or the adult equivalents of non-earning members, mainly children) and higher economic dependency ratios (i.e. 'dependent CUs'/'total CUs') than other households, as shown by Table 3.1. Total household income per CU was significantly ($P<0.05$) inversely related to the number of household members ($r=-0.30$) and the economic dependency ratio ($r=-0.27$). Relatively large household sizes with a high degree of dependence were characteristics of poverty in this community.

3.2.3 Demographic Characteristics

The overall distribution of the study population, disaggregated by age and sex is illustrated in Table 3.2. The overall sex ratio was fairly even - 182 males to 176 females. It was noticeably masculinised for infants, and feminised for the over forty year olds. This will be discussed further in section 4.10.

3.2.4 Division of Productive Labour

A full seasonal activity calendar highlighting the gender division of productive labour is presented in Table 3.3. In summer, the main

TABLE 3.1 : HOUSEHOLD DEMOGRAPHY AND PRODUCTION

VARIABLE	INCOME GROUP MEANS (SD) 1	2	3	F	P
Household members	4.8 (1.4)	5.8 (1.3)	5.8 (1.7)	2.8	0.07
Dependent CUs	1.4 (0.8)	1.8 (0.8)	2.1 (1.0)	3.5	0.04
Economic Dependency Ratio (CUs)	.36 (.15)	.43 (.15)	.50 (.13)	3.4	0.04
Cultivated acreages : Paddy	2.6 (0.9)	2.1 (0.9)	1.0 (0.6)	16.1	0.00
Maize*	1.7 (1.5)	1.0 (1.2)	0.3 (0.5)	5.1	0.01
Sorghum*	1.5 (2.1)	1.1 (1.3)	0.8 (1.0)	1.0	0.37
Standardised acreage per CU	1.1 (0.3)	0.7 (0.2)	0.3 (0.2)	35.8	0.00
Total asset value per CU (`000 Rs.)*	15.6(5.3)	9.8 (3.3)	5.1 (2.6)	30.9	0.00
Yields (qu.):Paddy	35.4(15.1)	26.2(9.5)	14.5(7.2)	14.2	0.00
Maize*	6.6 (4.2)	3.6(2.5)	2.4(0.8)	4.9	0.01
Total produce value per CU (`00 Rs.)*	17.7 (5.7)	10.2(2.3)	5.0(2.4)	44.3	0.00

TABLE 3.2 : AGE DISTRIBUTION

AGE	MALE	FEMALE
< 12 months	25	17
12-23 months	12	12
24-60 months	25	21
5-9 years	23	28
10-14 years	14	13
15-40 years	70	67
> 40 years	13	20
Total :	182	176

TABLE 3.3 : ACTIVITY CALENDAR WITH GENDER DIVISION OF LABOUR
(M = male; F = female)

Month (festival)	Major activities		Rain (mm)
March (Holi)	Well/tank repairs (MF) Migrant labour (M)	Mahua flower/fruit, tamarind collection (F)	3.8
April (Ugadi)	Manuring (M)		12.6
May		Bidi-leaf picking (MF)	50.7
June	Ploughing (dry, then wet land) (M) Maize sowing (F)	Paddy sowing (F)	99.3
July	Maize weeding (F)	Paddy transplanting (F)	185.1
August	Fishing (M)	Fertiliser application (M) Paddy weeding (F)	169.6
September		Water regulation (M) Pesticide application (M)	158.3
October (Dussera)	Maize harvest (F) Sorghum sowing (F) (vegetables)	Paddy crop-guarding (M)	64.0
November (Deepavalli)		Paddy harvest (MF) Stacking and drying (M)	5.1
December	Sorghum guarding (MF)	Threshing (M) Winnowing (F)	4.9
January (Sankranti)	Sorghum harvest (MF)	Bagging/haulage (MF) Loan repayment (M)	0.8
February (Shivarathri)			1.7

activities are minor forest produce gathering, local non-agricultural and migrant labour, and land preparation. Dryland crops are sown first with the onset of the rains in mid-June, and these are the particular responsibility of women once the men have ploughed the land. Women are also heavily involved in paddy cultivation, particularly in July and August (transplanting and weeding) and November and December (harvesting and winnowing).

3.3 HOME PRODUCTION PROCESS

3.3.1 Labour Participation

Members of landed households generally worked on their own land and labour was not employed to the exclusion of family labour. The level and seasonality of unwaged (or on-farm) labour participation for men and women is shown in Table 3.4 and Figure 3.1. The average annual on-farm labour input of both men and women was significantly greater for the richer households ($P<0.01$). This held for each season except summer for women. Unwaged labour participation was highest in the rainy season and winter, when men worked relatively more on their own land than women, who were more active as agricultural labourers. The need for poorer households to supplement their income by hiring out individuals as agricultural labourers, particularly in the rains, often meant that sowing, transplanting or harvesting their plots is delayed until the optimum time had passed; female paddy transplanting gangs in the study area always started work on the larger irrigated landholdings.

3.3.2 Crop Production

The predominance of paddy is emphasised by considering crop yields. A significant gradient existed between income groups with respect to the mean household yields of both paddy and maize (see Table 3.1). The composite index, total value of household produce per CU gave the highest degree of association ($r=0.83$; $P<0.01$) with total household income per CU, of any socio- economic variable investigated, showing the particularly high proportion of household income derived from home production.

FIGURE 3.1 : SEASONAL ADULT LABOUR PARTICIPATION PROFILF

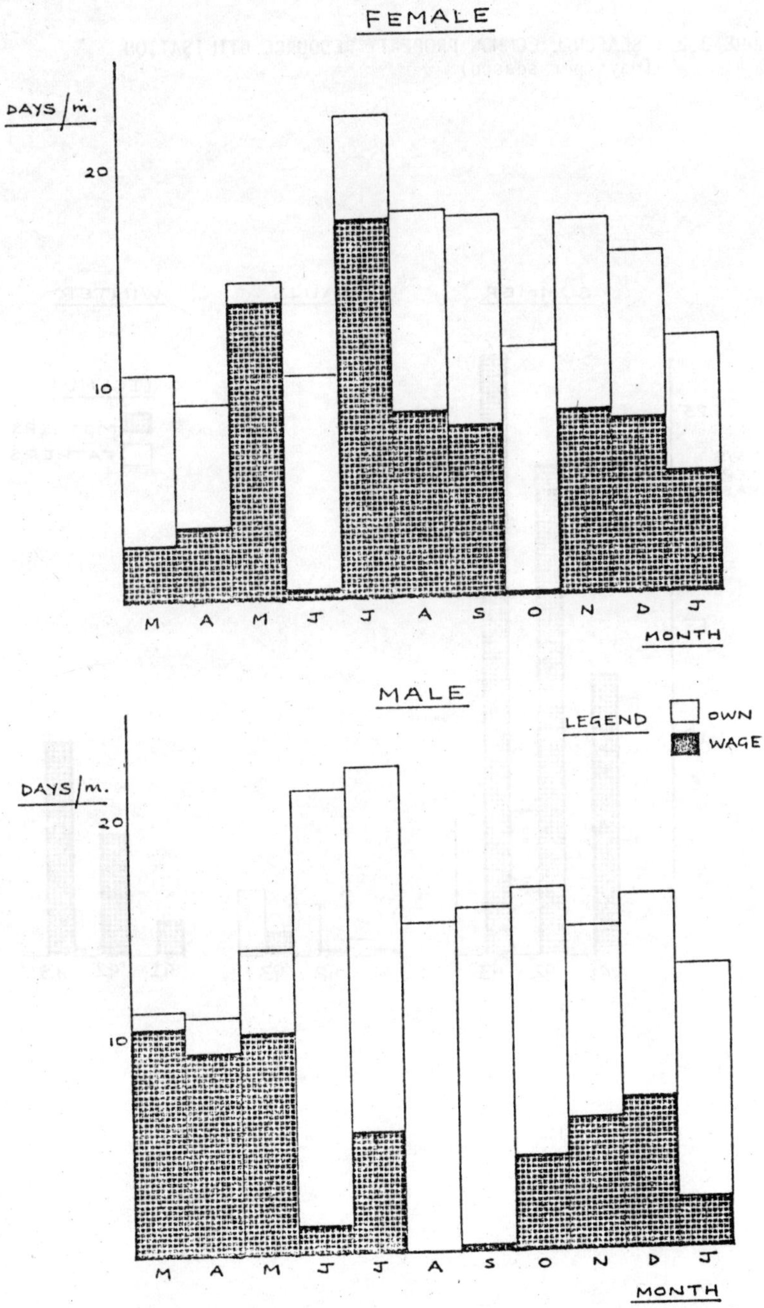

FIGURE 3.2 : SEASONAL COMMON PROPERTY RESOURCE UTILISATION
(days per season)

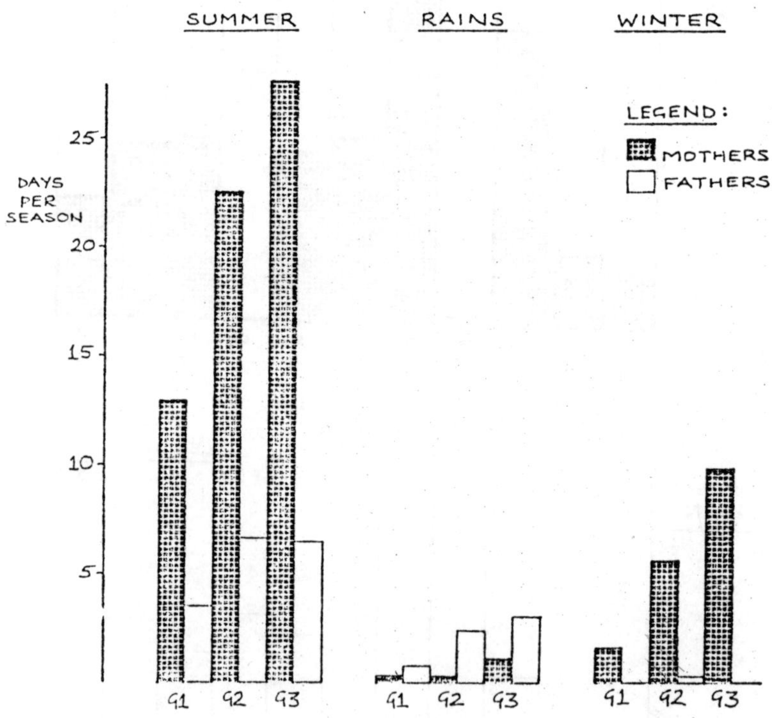

TABLE 3.4 : SEASONAL LABOUR PARTICIPATION IN WAGED AND OWN LABOUR (days/month) (M=male; F=female)

VARIABLE	INCOME GROUP MEANS (SD) 1	2	3	F	P
Summer :					
Own M	2.3 (2.6)	2.3 (2.8)	1.8 (3.1)	0.2	0.82
Own F	4.3 (2.2)	4.9 (3.6)	5.2 (3.0)	0.3	0.71
Wage M	7.9 (3.8)	10.5 (5.4)	11.1 (5.0)	1.8	0.18
Wage F	4.4 (3.9)	7.4 (5.2)	7.3 (3.7)	2.5	0.09
Rains :					
Own M	18.7 (2.9)	17.1 (2.0)	15.0 (3.6)	5.8	0.01
Own F	10.8 (3.5)	9.7 (2.5)	5.7 (3.4)	13.5	0.00
Wage M	0.8 (1.0)	1.7 (1.5)	2.8 (1.8)	6.7	0.00
Wage F	6.2 (3.2)	8.8 (3.3)	10.7 (4.6)	4.5	0.02
Winter :					
Own M	12.5 (2.8)	10.6 (3.0)	7.3 (3.1)	12.3	0.00
Own F	9.6 (3.9)	9.0 (2.9)	6.8 (2.5)	4.0	0.02
Wage M	2.3 (2.0)	5.0 (3.4)	7.6 (2.9)	11.9	0.00
Wage F	3.3 (2.9)	5.5 (3.6)	7.8 (2.8)	7.8	0.00

3.4 WAGE PRODUCTION PROCESS

3.4.1 Labour Participation

The mean monthly levels of waged (and unwaged) work for men and women are illustrated in Figure 3.1. For women, waged labour peaks occurred in the rains (sowing, transplanting, weeding) and during the bidi-leaf picking season in May, while male waged labour was at its highest level in summer. Women hired themselves out throughout the year, while only men from poorer households engaged in waged work to any extent in the rainy season. Aggregating waged and unwaged labour, peaks occurred for men and women in the rains (particularly July), and troughs in summer, after the harvest.

Examining socio-economic differences, in poorer households male and female hire-out peaked in the rains and winter i.e. the agricultural season, and was significantly higher, in terms of days wage labour per month ($P<0.01$) for these households in these seasons. There were no socio-economic differences in wage labour participation in summer. For each income group, women worked proportionately more wage, than on-farm, labour days than did men. (For example, in the richest Group 1, 36% total days worked by women were wage labour, as compared to 24% for men. In the poorest Group 3, the proportions were 60% and 40% for women and men respectively.) In terms of the aggregate (waged and unwaged) labour participation, however, income-group differences were not significant for men or women in any season, except summer for women.

3.4.2 Common Property Resource Utilisation

The total number of days spent by men and women in gathering minor forest produce, whether for sale or home consumption, are shown for each season in Figure 3.2. Summer was the most important season, when many forest fruits ripened and bidi leaves were picked for piece-rate wages from non-tribal contractors. This type of activity virtually ceased during the rains. Women, particularly from poor households, participated more than men. In summer, for example, G3 women spent on average the equivalent of nearly one month collecting forest produce, as compared to about one week for G3 men. Socio-economic differences were significant for each season for women

(P<0.05), but not men.

3.4.3 Wage Rates

The daily wage rates for men and women for different tasks and the modes of payment are given in Table 3.5. The division of labour in agriculture was quite marked, and paddy harvesting was the only activity in which both men and women participated (and received the same daily wage). In general, however, the lower paid tasks were carried out by women, who also received lower wages than men for some non-agricultural work.

3.4.4 Individuals' Income

Sources

Parental income earned from various sources is shown in Figure 3.3 which gives the percentage breakdown of total individuals' income by source for each income group. In absolute terms, both men and women in poorer households earned significantly more than their counterparts in richer households from agricultural labour (kind) (P<0.01), local non-agricultural work (P<0.05) and minor forest produce gathering (P<0.05). In relative terms, the latter provides a small proportion of total household income, but it virtually all accrued in the late summer months of April and May (see Figure 3.2), when it was the only source of income for some families.

Unlike men, there were no marked socio-economic differences in cash-paid agricultural labour for women. This was due to the fact that most women, irrespective of income group, participated in paddy transplanting - the predominant cash income source - generally as gang-labour.

Lambadi men earned significantly more than Koya men from migrant work, particularly in the summer. This was usually construction work on building sites in Warangal or Hanamakonda, where Lambadis have traditionally constituted a large part of the labour force for such work. Koyas, on the other hand, tended to remain in the forest more in summer, and earn relatively more than Lambadis from local non-agricultural work, such as repairing tanks, digging wells, etc.

Annually, women earned more than twice the cash income from

agricultural labour and minor forest produce gathering than did men. Men earned twice as much as women from local non-agricultural labour and much more from migrant labour, a source from which few women earned income. The tendency for men temporarily to migrate in search of work may be contributing to the feminisation of the agricultural labour force (a phenomenon that has also been observed in recent village studies carried out in Tamil Nadu (see Harriss 1987b)).

Levels of aggregated individual labour income earned by men and women were comparable. Men earned more on average than women in G1 and G3; less in G2. There were no significant socio-economic differences for men, but G2 and G3 women earned significantly more ($P<0.05$) than G1 women. Women from some of the richest households in G1 may be able to voluntarily withdraw from the wage labour force at certain times of the year.

Seasonality

The seasonality of income earned is illustrated in Figure 3.4 which shows seasonal mean monthly income values for men and women. Women earned more in the rains than in the summer or winter. There was a marked seasonality of income-earning with over one third of total income being earned in one month, July, through paddy transplanting. Payment of wages, however, was often delayed until cash was more readily available. It was not uncommon for women to have to wait until September, after the maize harvest, to receive payment for transplanting work carried out in July. Another peak occurred in May, when the women were bidi leaf picking.

Men, by contrast, had their highest levels of mean monthly income in summer, and their lowest in the rains. There was less seasonality in income-earning than with women. The relatively high mean monthly incomes from March to May were largely due to those men who migrate in search of work. There were other peaks in July (ploughing) and December (paddy harvesting).

TABLE 3.5 : DAILY LABOUR WAGE RATES FOR MEN AND WOMEN (2)

TASK	DAILY WAGE (Rs) MEN	WOMEN
Ploughing ; wet land with own bullocks	20	-
without bullocks	15	-
dry land with own bullocks	15	-
without bullocks	10	-
Sowing	-	10
Paddy transplanting (usually contract basis)	-	8 or 120/acre
Weeding	-	5
Harvesting ; maize and sorghum (in kind)	-	9
paddy (in kind)	9	9
Rolling and tying sheaves (in kind)	-	10
Stacking sheaves (in kind)	12	-
Threshing (in kind)	15	-
Winnowing (in kind)	-	9
Well-digging	10	7
Tank-repairing	8	5
Urban construction work	15	10
Bidi leaf picking (1 Rs./500 leaves)	10-15	10-15

FIGURE 3.3 : SOURCES OF INDIVIDUAL ADULT INCOME (%)

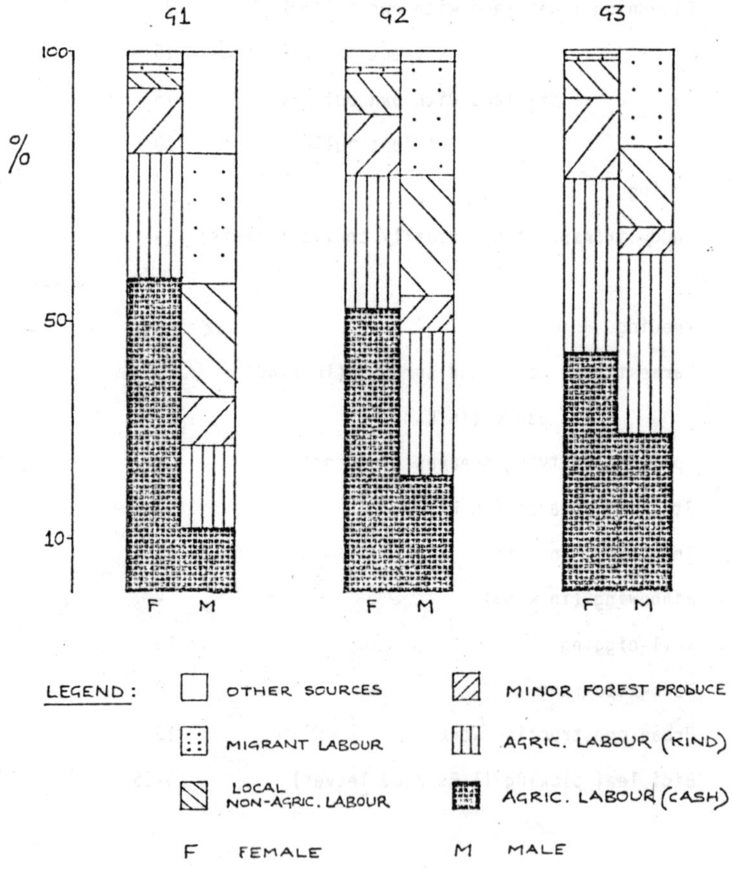

FIGURE 3.4 : SEASONALITY OF INDIVIDUAL ADULT INCOME

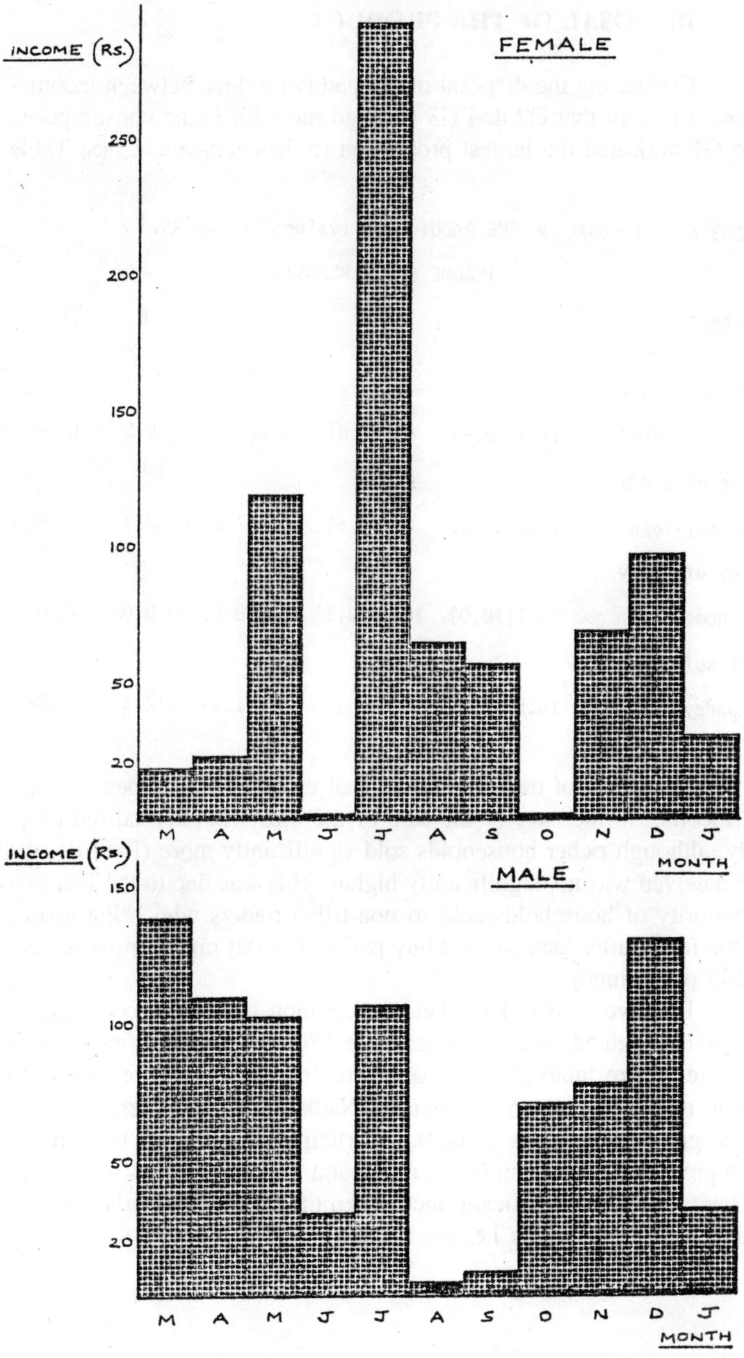

3.5 DISPOSAL OF THE PRODUCT

Comparing the disposal of the paddy produce between income-groups, it is seen that G2 and G3 retained most for home consumption, while G1 allocated the largest proportion to debt repayment (see Table 3.6).

TABLE 3.6 : DISPOSAL OF THE PADDY CROP (values in '00 Rs.)

VARIABLE	INCOME GROUP MEANS(SD) 1	2	3	F	P
Value of paddy sold*	11.7(10.9)	8.5(7.8)	1.9(4.3)	6.2	0.00
Value of paddy to repay loan*	17.1(13.0)	8.8(6.8)	3.8(7.6)	9.3	0.00
Value of paddy for home	23.1(10.0)	20.3(10.1)	12.8(8.6)	5.0	0.01
Self-sufficiency in paddy (months)	10.5 (2.9)	7.8(3.1)	5.3(1.9)	12.5	0.00

The terms of trade for the sale of crops did not appear to vary with income. In the case of the sale of the most commercialised crop, paddy, although richer households sold significantly more (P<0.01), the price received was not significantly higher. This was due to the fact that the majority of households sold to non-tribal traders who bring lorries into the forest after harvest, and buy paddy at a flat rate (approximately Rs. 145 per quintal).

Relative levels of market participation for each income-group may be investigated by examining Table 3.6. Nadkarni's definition was used here, where 'market participation' or 'commercialisation' refers to the sale of produce on to the market (Nadkarni 1980). There were no income-group differences in market participation - only 5 households which produced grain (1 in G1, 2 in G2 and 2 in G3) did not sell any of it. There were no significant income-group differences either in the relative marketed surplus i.e. the proportion of total grain sold (using mean prices for each group) to that produced - percentages ranged from 32.4% and 31.1% for G1 and G2, to 21.2% for G3.

Although prices received for paddy sale did not differ much between groups (ranging from 142-148 Rs./quintal), there were differences in the motives behind market involvement. G3 households, who were very dependent on the market for food purchases (see 3.8.1) generally sold to enable whole or partial repayment of loans before the post-Sankranti interest rate increase. For this income-group, marketable surplus was less than marketed surplus i.e. their apparent surplus was not actually surplus to their consumption requirements - a type of involvement that has been found to exist in other rainfed areas of South India (Gillespie 1983; Harriss 1983).

By contrast, G1 households were not nearly so market-dependent. They retained sufficient paddy to last most of the year, but still made post-harvest sales at the standard trader's rate, as a high percentage of the returns were used to repay the large loans taken, for example, to increase irrigation. The richest households in G1, as shown in Table 3.7, had the highest degree of absolute indebtedness, and recent productive investments having yet not made substantial returns, they were not in a sufficiently financially stable position to be able to speculate and hoard, unlike non-tribal moneylenders.

3.6 DISTRIBUTION OF INCOME

3.6.1 Poverty

The prevalence and intensity of poverty in the study population were examined by evaluating income distributions against national and local poverty lines. The distribution of total household income per CU has been shown in Figure 1.2.

Using the annual national poverty line and applying it to 70% of per capita household income, 88.1% households were found to be below the line (i.e. 59 of the 67). This was higher than the 1985 average for Telengana of 60%, as reported by Shatrugna (1985). This percentage corresponds to the 'head-count' measure, H, referred to by Sen (1981) and fails to capture the intensity of poverty of those households who lie below the line. Sen suggests the use of another measure - the 'income gap ratio', I, which is the percentage short- fall of the average income of the 'poor' from the poverty line. In this study population, I=0.68. The average per capita income as a multiple of the poverty line was 0.75, ranging from 0.32 to 1.67. Given that gross, and not net, income is being considered here, it is unlikely that any household in this community would have had an investible surplus, according to the national line.

Using the local poverty line, 25.4% households (17 of the 67) were below the line i.e. had 70% household income per CU values less than Rs. 818. This was a much lower proportion than that obtained with the adjusted national line, and compared with the figure of 15% households below a local poverty line, derived in a similar fashion, for Golloor, a village in Hyderabad District of Andhra Pradesh in 1978-79 agricultural year (Shears 1982), although this used net, as opposed to gross income. In the latter study, 81% households were below the national poverty line, as compared to 88.1% in this study. The income gap ratio of the 'poor', I was 0.87. The mean per CU income as a poverty line multiple was 1.34, ranging from 0.59 to 3.23.

Comparisons of the local and national poverty lines highlight very distinctly the problems that arise from using average national statistics to measure the extent of local poverty. The local line was more specific in identifying potential target groups than the national line which was not very meaningful in operational terms.

3.6.2 Ultra Poverty

In this study population, 10 out of 67 households (15%) were defined as being 'ultra poor' by the 'double 80' rule. This fell in line with Lipton's estimate of 10-20% of low income country households being 'ultra poor'. Although 8 of the 17 households below the local poverty line (i.e. in G3) were 'ultra poor', food behavioural characteristics here cannot be assumed to be directly and closely associated with poverty, when the other 2 'ultra poor' households came from the richest income group, G3.

It should be noted that the measures investigated up to this point relate to numerical definitions of poverty, and as Chambers (1987) has stated: "Lipton may have pushed analysis of statistics about as far as it can go, with his poor and ultra-poor. The next breakthroughs may come through identifying relationships which statistics do not reveal or have not yet caught up with, and most of all through learning the priorities and criteria of well-being from poor people themselves".

3.6.3 Inequality

The income and asset value shares were as follows :

Income per CU: top 20% owned 30%
bottom 20% owned 12%

Asset value: top 20% owned 38%
per CU bottom 20% owned 7%

The Lorenz curve for total household income per CU was plotted and is shown in Figure 3.5. The Gini coefficients (G) were as follows

- total household income (G=0.205)
- total household income per CU (G=0.154)
- total household asset value (G=0.284)
- total household asset value per CU (G=0.290)

The coefficients had exceptionally low values for agrarian societies, indicating a relatively high degree of equality of income and asset distribution in this study population. The asset value coefficient was higher, largely because of the influence of land value, particularly wetland, which amplified the slight inequality in income distribution. The degree to which the differentiation in this community has been brought about by cyclical demographic processes, as opposed to economic processes, is investigated in Appendix V.

Comparing these results with those obtained using data collected in 1978-79 from two non-tribal villages, Golloor and Sahebnagar, in Hyderabad District and cited by Harriss (1983), they were seen to be considerably lower. Gini coefficients for household land value and total per capita income had values of 0.42 and 0.31 (Golloor) and 0.50 and 0.34 (Sahebnagar). Corbridge (1986) calculated a Gini coefficient of 0.41 for land use in the tribal Jharkhand region of Bihar.

FIGURE 3.5 : LORENZ CURVE OF TOTAL INCOME PER CU

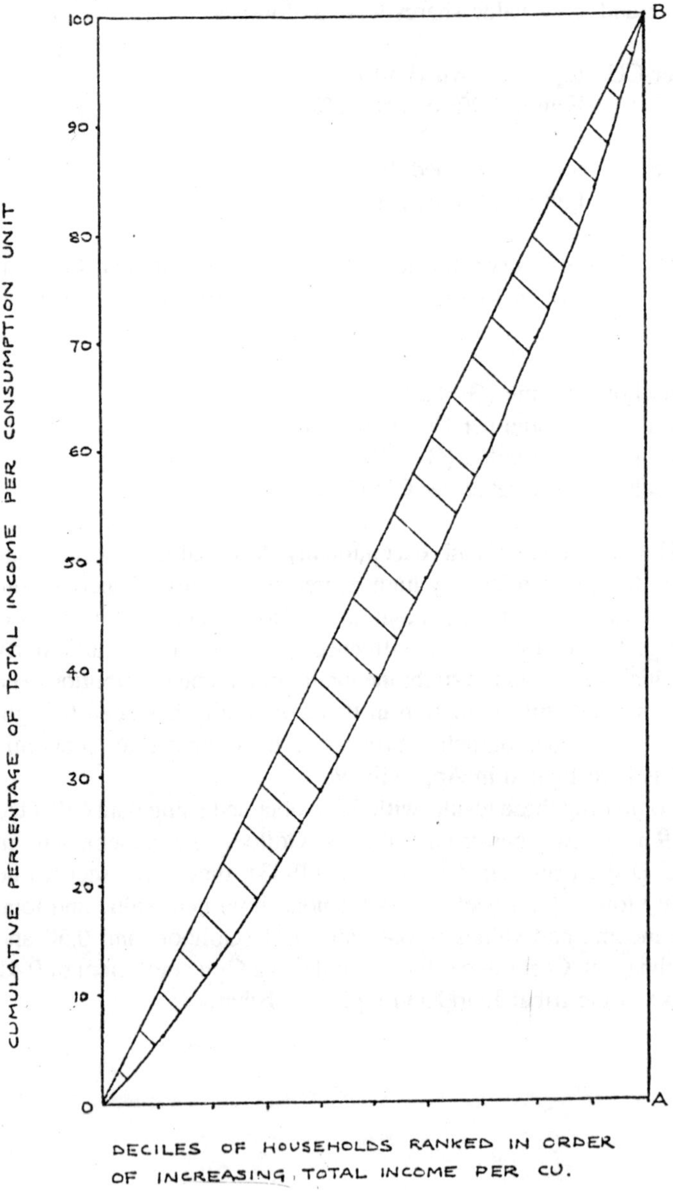

3.7 CREDIT AND DEBT

The great majority of loans were taken at the beginning of the agricultural year in June or July, in order to purchase agricultural inputs such as fertilisers, pesticides, herbicides (and maybe even seeds), and pay hired-in labour. There were no income-group differences in the number of loans taken with each study household having taken on average two major loans in the 1985-86 agricultural year. Involvement in the market for credit was nearly universal with only one household in the study not having taken a loan.

In terms of the total loan per CU, the G1 mean was over twice those of G2 and G3 (P<0.01), which were of a similar magnitude (see Table 3.7). Loans from private sources were much larger than those from banks for each group. 84% households took private loans, as compared to only 49% which took bank loans.

The mean percentage of total loan to total income for G1 and G3 were virtually equal at about 38%, with G2 at 28% This ratio has been suggested as an index of financial precariousness (Watson 1984). This would seem, however, to presuppose similar uses for loans contracted. The large G1 value here was largely due to the long-term investment by several households in productive assets e.g. motor-driven water pumps to increase irrigation, whereas a much higher proportion of G3 loans were used for consumption purposes. Absolute and relative indebtedness were not characteristics of poverty in this study.

TABLE 3.7 : MONEY MARKET OPERATION

VARIABLE	INCOME GROUP MEANS (SD) 1	2	3	F	P
Loans ('00 Rs.) :					
Bank*	9.0(10.5)	5.8(7.7)	1.4(2.8)	3.8	0.03
Private	12.9 (9.1)	10.0(8.6)	11.8(8.5)	0.6	0.54
Total per CU*	8.9 (7.6)	4.2(2.3)	3.7(2.6)	4.5	0.02
Loan to total income ratio (%)	37.7(24.2)	28.0(14.7)	37.8(27.6)	1.7	0.19

The money market did not discriminate directly against the poorest borrowers in terms of interest rates - there were no significant income-group differences in six monthly interest rates for either bank or private loans. The average interest rate on private loans (41%) was about four times that on bank loans (10%) and these rates applied to each group.

The discrimination that did exist was of a different type. 75% G3 households, as compared to 50% in G2 and only 31% in G1 did not take out bank loans. Poorer households owned less land and were less likely to have land title deeds (or 'pattas'), having obtained relatively more land through officially illegal encroachment on the forest. As 'pattas' were necessary collateral on a bank loan , those households without them were not eligible. There was therefore less direct access by the poorest households to institutional credit which had the lowest interest rate. This type of discrimination has been documented elsewhere in South India (Watson and Harriss 1985; Prasad *et al.* 1986; Ramachandran 1986)

Private moneylenders, despite the higher interest rates charged were generally turned to for loans for several reasons :

- collateral or security was not required. Defaulting was uncommon due to social pressures - moneylenders colluded over information on past defaulters, and the latter would find it very difficult to obtain loans in the same area in the future,
- unlike banks, money could be used for any purpose, (A certain proportion of a bank loan would have to be used for a stipulated purpose, e.g. to purchase fertiliser. The receipts from this transaction would then need to be produced at the bank before the remainder of the loan was made available.),
- less bureaucracy and paperwork was required. The debtor need not be literate,
- money was readily available without a time lag between application and availability, (To reduce this lag, borrowers might bribe bank officials.)
- the trader-moneylender was accessible throughout the day and night,
- relative flexibility of repayment procedures. Normally repayment was in kind after the harvest.

For many of these reasons, richer households took, on average, larger loans from private than from institutional sources. If the debt was not discharged after six months, the interest rate increased. High interest rates were disguised by the interlocking of money and food markets. If a loan was taken in July, then it was usually required to be repaid six months later at harvest time (Sankranti) with interest of 3 kunsums paddy per Rs. 100 loan (1 kunsum = 11 kg. paddy) i.e. a rate of approximately 42% per six months. The informal credit market was thus entrenched in both household production and consumption.

The moneylender may be able to speculate, hoarding paddy and selling months later during the monsoon at higher prices, at a time when transport to fair-price shops was difficult. He may also take advantage of economies of scale with transport costs and, bypassing middlemen, sell later in bulk at outside markets.

Informal inter-household loans of small quantities of paddy, without interest, were made occasionally. This type of loan was more common between relatives during the rainy season to tie families over until they could either afford the time and/or cash to visit the fair-price shop in Kothaguddem and buy rice in bulk.

3.8 EFFECTIVE DEMAND - DISPOSAL OF NET INCOME

The mean monthly cash expenditures per CU on different foodstuffs, liquor and tobacco and health for each income group, in each season are given in Table 3.8. Income-group differences were generally most significant in summer, when poorer households' food stocks were dwindling (see 3.9.1) and they were becoming more dependent on the market for staple food purchases (see Figure 3.6), while cutting back on expenditure on more expensive foods and liquor. The paddy harvest had a levelling influence on these income differences, which were consequently least in winter.

3.8.1 Staples

The seasonal trends in market dependence for staples across income-groups are illustrated in Figure 3.6. 'Market dependence' here refers to the purchase of commodities from the market (Nadkarni 1980). As argued by Harriss (1983), an increasing dependence on the vagaries of market exchange is likely to be associated both with poverty and with nutritionally inadequate control over grain.

The extent of market dependence was greatest in summer and least in winter, when no G1 household was market-dependent. Chi-Squared analyses (3) show income-group differences in market dependence to have been significant in the summer (Chi sq.=19.6; 2 d.f.; P<0.001) and the rains (Chi sq.=18.3; 2 d.f.; P<0.001) when approximately 90% G3 households were market-dependent, but not in winter (Chi sq.=4.3; 2 d.f.;P>0.1). As shown in Table 3.6, G1 households had household food stocks sufficient for 10.5 months, on average, according to the household head, as compared to 7.8 months for G2 and 5.3 months for G3 households.

FIGURE 3.6 : SEASONALITY OF STAPLE FOOD MARKET DEPENDENCE

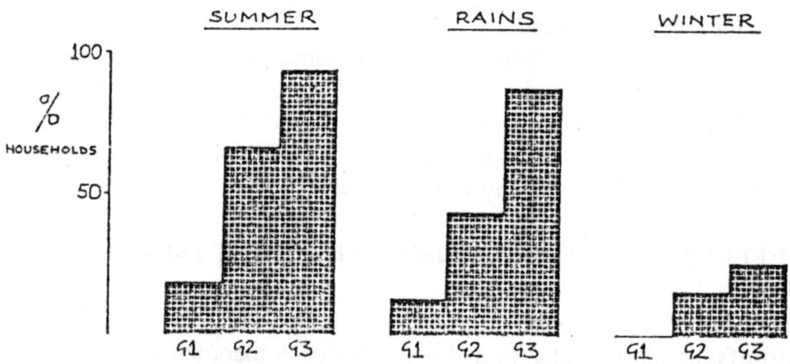

With regard to the terms of trade for the purchase of commodities, the vast majority of households which were not self-sufficient, bought staples from the government-controlled fair-price shop in Kothaguddem at fixed rates (approximately Rs. 2.2 per kg. rice).

The proportion of grain purchased to that produced was significantly (P<0.01) higher in the poorer households, as was the proportion purchased to that sold (P<0.01), which gives another indication of the socio-economic differences in the relative degree and type of involvement in the market. Groups 1 and 2 both purchased less than half the quantity of grain that they sold (G1, only 5%), whereas G3 bought nearly twice as much as it sold. This corroborates Hill's finding that the richer cultivators are the only real subsistence farmers (Hill 1980).

3.8.2 Other Foods

Vegetables and meat. Richer households spent significantly more in these two categories (P<0.05), except meat in winter (P=0.08).

For the richest group, G1, there were no marked seasonal differences in expenditure, while G2 and G3 spent significantly more on both vegetables and meat in winter than in summer or the rains.

TABLE 3.8 : MEAN MONTHLY EXPENDITURE PER CU ON FOOD AND HEALTH (Rs.)

VARIABLE		INCOME GROUP MEANS (SD)				
		1	2	3	F	P
Pulses	Summer	8.5(7.7)	8.6(9.9)	10.0(7.7)	0.2	0.83
	Rains	7.7(7.2)	6.0(6.8)	5.4(6.0)	0.5	0.59
	Winter	5.9(6.3)	3.5(6.1)	3.9(4.9)	0.9	0.42
Vegetables	Summer	32.3(11.8)	19.5(10.8)	14.4(8.8)	15.1	0.00
	Rains	29.0(12.2)	19.5 (8.1)	16.2(7.8)	9.4	0.00
	Winter	38.7(12.5)	30.1(10.8)	27.1(9.5)	5.1	0.01
Meat	Summer	21.4(13.2)	10.6 (9.1)	4.0 (6.8)	13.0	0.00
	Rains	21.2 (8.6)	14.9 (8.8)	9.2 (9.2)	7.4	0.00
	Winter	24.1 (9.0)	21.8(10.2)	16.1(11.4)	2.6	0.08
Spices/oil	Summer	21.8 (6.4)	17.0 (4.1)	15.1 (3.3)	8.8	0.00
	Rains	21.3 (6.0)	16.8 (4.2)	14.6 (3.2)	9.5	0.00
	Winter	23.1 (6.1)	22.6 (7.0)	18.8 (4.8)	2.4	0.10
Liquor/ tobacco	Summer	28.8 (9.2)	18.1 (8.6)	11.8 (9.4)	14.8	0.00
	Rains	28.7 (8.8)	19.1 (8.4)	14.1 (8.3)	12.4	0.00
	Winter	30.4 (7.8)	25.3(10.4)	17.4(11.0)	7.0	0.00
Health	Summer	21.9 (8.4)	15.4 (5.6)	10.4 (9.4)	9.8	0.00
	Rains	20.3 (7.2)	13.4 (8.0)	12.4 (5.2)	6.3	0.00
	Winter	21.4 (7.5)	17.8 (7.2)	16.8 (5.8)	2.0	0.15

Pulses. There was no significant income or seasonal effect, although noticeably more pulses were bought in summer than in the rains or winter.

Spices and oil. Richer households spent more for each season, though differences were only significant (P<0.01) in summer and the rains. There were no significant seasonal differences for any income group.

Overall food. There was no significant income or seasonal effect.

Liquor and tobacco. Richer households spent significantly more (P<0.01) for each season, and, again, there were no marked seasonal changes.

3.8.3 Health

Richer households spent more in each season, though this was only significant in summer and the rains. There were no significant seasonal changes for any income group. The relationship between the seasonality of health expenditure and child morbidity is fully investigated in section 4.9.

3.8.4. Food Behaviour

Engel's Law was seen to operate overall; as income per CU increased, the proportion spent on food declined. Regressing the proportion of income spent on food per CU against total income per CU, gave a significant (P<0.01) inverse relationship (r=-0.63). However, logging the proportion and re-regressing gave a higher degree of association (r=-0.66), showing that the relationship was likely to be a curved one. 56% of the association though was still unexplained.

The 'ultra poor' households as a group did, in fact, flout this law, inasmuch as the correlation coefficient (r=-0.37) for the association between the logged proportion and total income per CU was insignificant (P=0.29), although only 10 households were included.

With regard to the 'law of starchy staples', it did not appear to apply in these villages. As income rose, there was no substitution of inferior staples by higher quality and/or higher priced staples. Rice consumption was virtually universal, and sorghum and maize, when consumed, did not substitute for, but supplemented rice in the diet.

3.9 REPRODUCTION OF THE CONSUMPTION UNIT

The forces, process and relations of household reproduction will be described in this section, with particular attention being given to the effect of household socio-economic status and seasonality on energy consumption and patterns of maternal time allocation.

3.9.1 Household Energy Consumption

There were seasonal changes, and socio-economic differences in the mean daily quantity of rice consumed per CU. Daily, most rice was consumed in the post-harvest winter months (overall mean : 0.79 kg. per CU); least in the rains (overall mean : 0.67 kg. per CU). For each season, the daily rice consumption per CU of richer households was significantly higher (P<0.01) than their poorer counterparts.

Sorghum was the second most commonly consumed staple with a maximum of 30% households in summer, and a minimum of 15% households in winter consuming it. Koyas rarely consumed sorghum in these villages, while in Lambadi households it is prepared as chappatis to supplement rice in the diet.

Maize was the least commonly consumed staple. It is either roasted on the cob ('kanki') or ground and consumed as a gruel ('ambali'). Only 10% households in summer and the rains, and no households in winter consumed it. As with sorghum, there were no significant mean income-group differences in daily quantities consumed per household.

The income-group mean household energy consumption levels (kcals. per CU) attained by staple food intake alone for each season are illustrated in Table 3.9. A negative gradient was observed from winter-to-summer-to-rains, for each income-group. Seasonally, there was little change for G1, but with G2 and G3, calories obtained per CU significantly increased from rains to winter (P<0.01) and decreased from winter to summer (P<0.05). There was also a significant (P<0.01) negative gradient from G1-G2-G3, for each season., particularly the rains.

In each season, the deficit was particularly marked for G3 , whose means were significantly lower than those for G1 and G2, as revealed by the Scheffe test. As pointed out in a prior section, male and female levels of physical work (in terms of mean monthly total days work), which may be taken as a rough proxy of energy expenditure, did not vary significantly between groups (see Table 3.4). However, the co-incidence of a particularly low level of household staple energy consumption for G3 households, with a period of general peak labour demand, in the rainy season was disturbing.

TABLE 3.9 : DAILY HOUSEHOLD ENERGY CONSUMPTION PER CU (KCALS./DAY)

	INCOME GROUP MEANS (SD)				
SEASON	1	2	3	F	P
Summer	2626(414)	2397(282)	2071(302)	13.5	0.00
Rains	2569(393)	2298(269)	1942(230)	18.1	0.00
Winter	2694(376)	2603(332)	2282(264)	7.3	0.00

These findings were compared with other S. Asian studies. In Bangladesh, Becker *et al.* (1986) found that the quantity of specific foods consumed by the household was positively related to household income. In other South Indian studies, however, the relationship between household income and calorie consumption has been found to be weak (Harriss 1987a). Bidinger *et al.* (1986) in a study in Andhra Pradesh, found there to be no relationship between household calorie consumption and income and no seasonal variation in the former due, they claimed, to the pattern of credit and (circular) debt and the reasonably stable food prices in the area.

In this study, however, although private moneylenders were readily available, it was not common for them to be regularly turned to for small consumption loans when the need arose. Rather, a portion of the large loan taken in the early rains was usually set aside for consumption purposes and rationed. Although food prices at the fair-price shop were generally stable, the shop was often out-of-stock and/or inaccessible, particularly in the rains when food stocks were beginning to run low in poorer households. The opportunity cost in terms of one days' income foregone to visit the shop, moreover, was particularly high for the poorer households.

Another factor probably contributing to the income and seasonal effect on foodgrain consumption was the omission by certain households at certain times (again usually the rains) of one meal during the day. These households were generally those more dependent on wage labour (i.e. the poorer households (see Table 3.4) due to the need to start wage labour particularly early in the day. This phenomenon has been observed elsewhere (Chimwaza 1982; Haaga and Mason 1987).

3.9.2 Adult Time Allocation

The time allocation of mothers and fathers of children under 24 months of age, in each group at three mid-seasonal points is illustrated in Figure 3.7. In terms of overall hours worked per day there was no significant difference between groups for either men or women, at the three seasonal points. Women overall worked more hours per day (11-12.5) than men (9-12). They also spent more time (5-6 hours) on 'domestic' activities, including child care, than men (1-2 hours).

There were inter-group differences in the type of work performed. Poorer households had higher ratios of hours spent on agricultural wage labour to own-farm labour. There were, however, no marked inter-group differences in the levels of total domestic work input for either men or women.

Seasonally, for men and women, the least number of hours' work per day was in the March survey. For men of each group, most daily hours work were recorded in July; for women, similar levels of time input were recorded in July and November.

Time allocated by women to 'child care' varied seasonally. For each group, women spent more time in summer on this activity, least in the rains. Time allocated to 'child care' by parents from the poorest households was generally least, probably due to the need for wage labourers to start work earlier than on-farm workers. Moreover, women from these households spent the most time on 'other domestic work' - a large proportion of which was water-fetching, their having no wells of their own, unlike richer households.

3.9.3 Household-level Decision-making

The distribution of married couples according to husband/wife involvement in various areas of household decision-making is shown in Table 3.10. In 45 percent households, men were the sole decision-makers in the three areas of expenditure on agricultural inputs, food and

FIGURE 3.7 : SEASONALITY OF PARENTAL TIME ALLOCATION

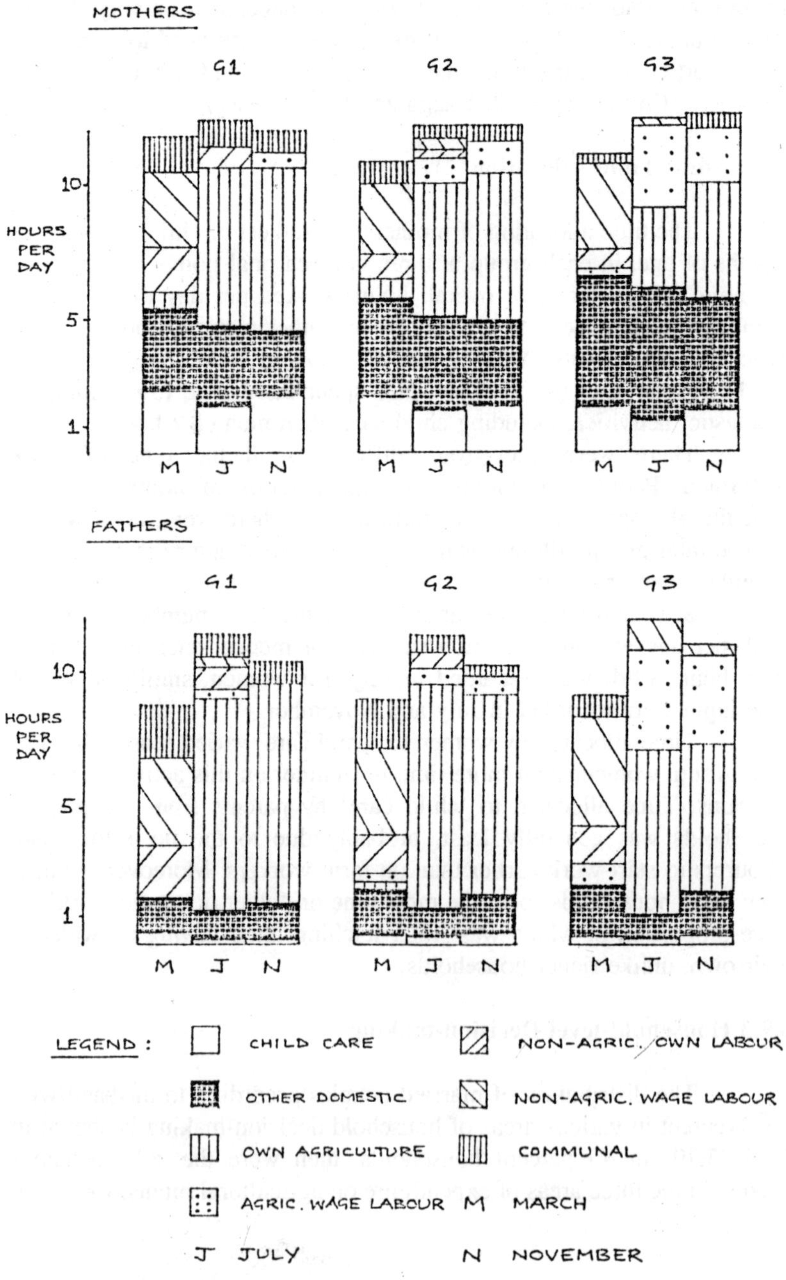

health. Men had greater decision-making power in matters relating to health than food, although even in the latter area, they were generally dominant.

TABLE 3.10 : PARENTAL DECISION-MAKING INVOLVEMENT

AREA OF DECISION-MAKING	DECISION MAKERS (% households)		
	SOLE MALE	JOINT	SOLE FEMALE
Agricultural inputs	95.5	4.5	-
Food expenditure	46.3	35.8	17.9
Health expenditure	80.5	10.5	9.0

In order to better understand the characteristics of households containing women who played an active role in decision-making, the study population was divided with respect to whether women, either solely or with men, were involved in making decisions relating to expenditure on food and/or health. T-tests were carried out to detect differences in means of various socio-economic variables between these two subsamples. The following socio-economic characteristics of 'female decision-making households' were statistically significant. The P values are shown in parentheses :

- high total income per CU from sale of labour (0.01)
- low amount total loan taken per CU (0.02)
- high male income per CU from migrant labour (0.03)

Disaggregating by income group, it emerges that in G2 and G3, 50-60% households contained women involved in decision-making, as compared to only 31% in G1. Anti-female bias was thus particularly evident in the richest households. Women were more involved in decision-making in the poorer households, dependent on the wage labour of both adult women and men; particularly those households containing men who migrated during the year to find work, leaving their wives at home. This would seem to corroborate evidence from other South Asian studies (Jeffrey *et al.* 1987) which has shown less gender bias in decision-making in asset-less or asset-poor households, where patrilineal control over property was least.

Households in which women were involved in decision-making were not those with higher relative female-to-male economic participation, as hypothesised by Bardhan (1985), although a high absolute level of female income was an associated characteristic. Recent South Asian studies have similar findings (see Harriss 1987a). Status may not be adequately defined by participation in the wage labour force. Cultural factors are likely to be important, including aspects of kinship such as age at marriage, resource transfers at marriage, control over dowry etc. (Caldwell and Caldwell 1987)

In this tribal area, womens' duties were generally associated closely with the collective family aspects of consumption, while men were much more individuated in relation to their control over resources, and in relation to their own consumption (e.g. liquor and tobacco). Income from wage work was categorised into different types of expenditure (e.g. collective consumption, household food budget, fund for consumer durables, etc.) and a division of responsibility as to these items between husband and wife existed, with the latter taking the major responsibility for matters concerning the household as a unity. The situation here was similar to those found in West Africa and Britain by Whitehead (1981) in her study of the politics of domestic budgetting.

Eka Venkatama of Ravenniguddem highlighted this when she spoke of the money she earns picking bidi leaves in summer: "It is vital for me to pick leaves for as many hours and as many days as I can. The money will go towards buying 'pappu' (redgram), and I'll try to save some to buy some clothes for the children at Ugaḍi".

3.10 SUMMARY

Despite low values for indices of inequality within the study community, there were socio-economic differences between richer and poorer households. The classificatory variable, income per consumption unit, has empirically differentiated households with respect to the effects of the market mechanisms of surplus appropriation that operate. Poorer households had larger families, higher economic dependency ratios and smaller landholdings. They were more dependent on labour markets for their income, food markets for their consumption and exploitative private moneylenders for credit. Women in poorer households were particularly involved in gathering minor forest produce, either for sale or home consumption. The potential for households to reproduce themselves was least for the poorest households.

With regard to household reproduction, daily household energy consumption for the poorest households was least for each season, and particularly low in the rains - a time when levels of maternal time allocated to child care were also relatively low. Women had little involvement in intra-household decision-making in matters regarding food and health.

Notes

1. F is the ratio of the between-groups mean square to the within-groups mean square, sometimes called the variance ratio. The mean square, or variance, equals the sum of squared deviations of the observations about the overall mean, divided by the degrees of freedom. P is the probability that the null hypothesis is incorrectly rejected and represents the level of statistical significance of the F ratio.

2. The exchange rates at the beginning and the end of the study period, for rupees to US dollars, and for US dollars to pound sterling were:

March 1985:	12.96 Rs./$	1.12 $/LGB
February 1986:	12.37 Rs./$	1.43 $/LGB

3. The Chi squared test examines the association between the row variable and the column variable of a contingency table, or, in other words, whether the distribution of individuals among the categories of one variable is independent of their distribution among the categories of the other.

4

NUTRITIONAL AND HEALTH OUTCOMES

A characterisation of child growth retardation and morbidity in the study population is carried out in this section, data being disaggregated by the age and sex of the child. Firstly, the prevalence, severity and seasonality of growth retardation in under five year old children, according to classifications involving three anthropometric indicators and both international and regional anthropometric standards, is described. Households are classified according to patterns of adult and child anthropometry at one seasonal point in the year, in an attempt to determine the type of nutritional problems affecting families at a household level, at a particularly critical time of the year.

Secondly, characteristics of child morbidity are examined. These include the nature, incidence and seasonality of diseases, particularly diarrhoea. Adult perceptions of seasonal family vulnerability to ill-health and the relationship between the seasonality of health expenditure and child morbidity are also investigated.

4.1 CHILD GROWTH RETARDATION

4.1.1 Overall Under-Fives

The percentages of under-five year old children (n=112) in each nutritional status category, with respect to their annual mean values of the three anthropometric indicators, are shown in Table 4.1. The Gomez weight-for-age (WA) and the Waterlow height-for-age (HA) and weight-for-height (WH) classifications were used, with NCHS standards (and NIN standards with WA), as described in section 2.2.4, in order to compare the results with those of other Indian studies.

Comparing these results with other Indian studies, the percentage of severe WA cases in this study (7.2%) was seen to be higher than the median incidence of 2.6% (but within the range of 1.1 to 20%) cited by Poleman (1981) where 32,000 children were studied in six surveys in India. Hanumantha Rao *et al.* (1974) in a study of the nutritional status of pre-school Koya Dora tribals in East Godavari District, A.P. found 11.5% severe WA cases, 59% 'moderate', 29.5% 'mild' and no children classified as 'normal'. In a more recent study of the health and nutritional status of tribals in Madhya Pradesh, undertaken by NIN (1986), percentages of severely WA malnourished under-fives ranged from 6.5 to 11.3 %. Results from this study are actually very similar to the state-wide percentages of 7.8% and 36.7% for 'severe' and 'moderate' malnutrition, collected by the National Nutrition Monitoring Bureau (1981).

If, however, weight-for-height were to be considered as being the most appropriate index of nutritional well-being, as it is by some (Seckler 1981) then there appears to be no severe cases and only 10.7% 'moderately' malnourished.

TABLE 4.1 : ANNUAL PREVALENCE AND SEVERITY OF GROWTH RETARDATION ACCORDING TO THREE ANTHROPOMETRIC CLASSIFICATIONS (% under-fives)

INDICATOR	DEGREE OF GROWTH RETARDATION			
	THIRD `severe`	SECOND `moderate`	FIRST `mild`	NORMAL
Weight-for-age (NCHS)	7.2	41.0	51.8	0.0
Weight-for-age (NIN)	1.8	17.4	60.6	20.2
Height-for-age (NCHS)	6.3	23.2	19.5	51.0
Weight-for-height (NCHS)	0.0	10.7	48.2	41.1

4.1.2 By Age and Sex

Of the 8 severely WA malnourished children, 6 were in the under 12m. and 2 in the 12-23 m. age group. This, along with the picture of growth faltering revealed by the individual growth curves in section 4.1.3, would seem to corroborate evidence from other studies (De Chavez *et al.* 1974; Nabarro 1984; Prasad *et al.* 1986) that have shown that children of weaning age are particularly vulnerable to malnutrition. Approximately 60% in the under 12 m. age group, and 50% within both the other age groups were in the second or third degree categories.

FIGURE 4.1 : AGE-SEX GROUP BREAKDOWN OF CHILD GROWTH RETARDATION ACCORDING TO THREE ANTHROPOMETRIC CLASSIFICATIONS

LEGEND : ■ BOYS ; □ GIRLS ; 3° Third degree 2° Second degree 1° First degree N Normal

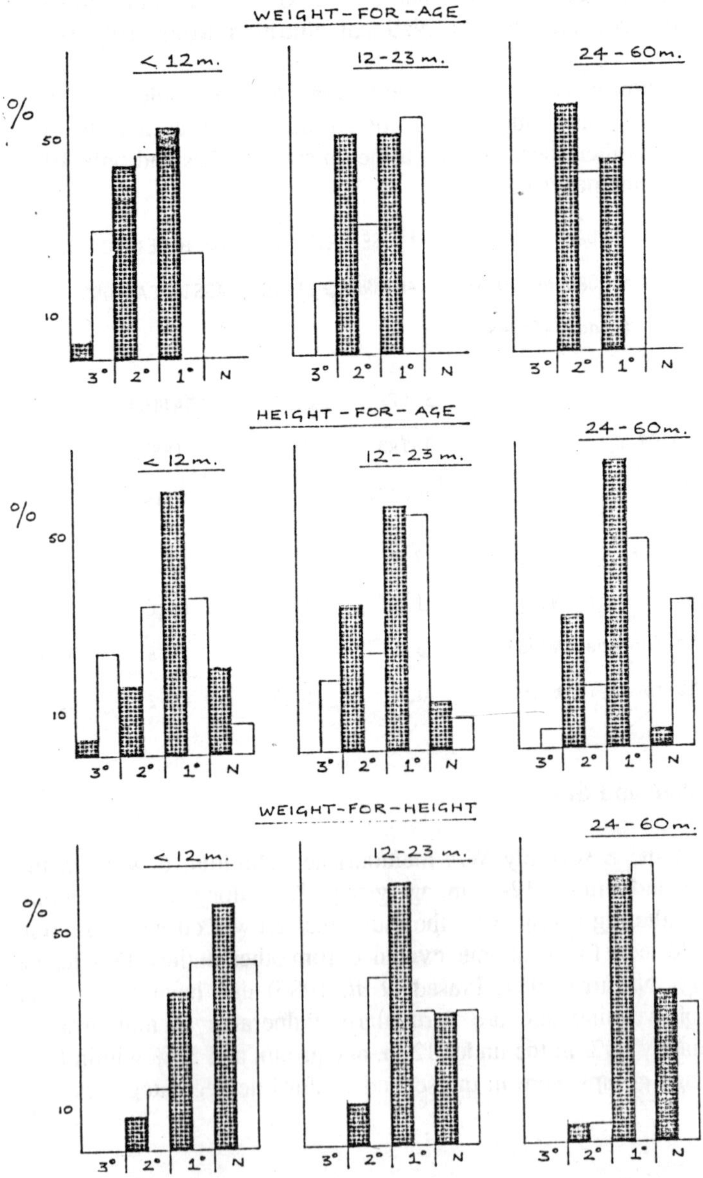

As regards the sex of the child, no fewer than seven of the eight severely WA malnourished children were girls. The percentages of study children within age-sex groups falling into each category are shown in Figure 4.1. Owing to the small cell numbers this gave, it was not possible to determine the statistical significance of any differences revealed.

29.4% girls under 12 months of age were severely WA malnourished (i.e. 5 out of 17), as compared to 4% (1 out of 25) boys in this age group. With the WA and HA indicators, as the child's age increased, higher proportions of boys and lower proportions of girls were in states of moderate or severe growth retardation. There were no severe WH cases, which indicates that severe malnutrition where it occurred was chronic, rather than acute.

Over the last five years, conflicting results regarding gender differences in child growth retardation have emerged. Studies in India, Nepal, Sri Lanka and Bangladesh have found no gender differences (Hilder and Steinhoff 1983; Martorell *et al.* 1984; Perera 1983; Abdullah 1983), while in two other studies in Bangladesh, (Chen *et al.* 1981; Bairagi 1983) significantly more under-five year old girls than boys were found to be severely malnourished.

Results from this study were most similar to those of Kynch and Maguire (1986), from a study in Uttar Pradesh, which showed that girls had a lower frequency distribution of anthropometric status than young boys and more frequent seasonal weight losses, but that there was a progressive decline in the status of boys vis-a-vis girls, with increasing age. Possible explanations for gender differences in infant nutritional status will be fully discussed in section 4.8, once the nutritional and morbidity profiles have been fully developed.

4.1.3 Growth Curves

Figure 4.2 shows individual growth curves for those boys and girls in the under 12 month age group along with the NCHS median and 60% NCHS median (i.e. severe malnutrition) curves. It should be recalled that any child aged under 12 months at the beginning of the study fell into the under 12 m. age group; hence some children in this group may have been as old as 23 months by the end of the study.

For the first four months of life, boys were seen to follow the NCHS median closely. Between 4-6 months, the growth rate started to

FIGURE 4.2 : INDIVIDUAL GROWTH CURVES OF UNDER 12 MONTH AGE GROUP CHILDREN, BY SEX

BOYS

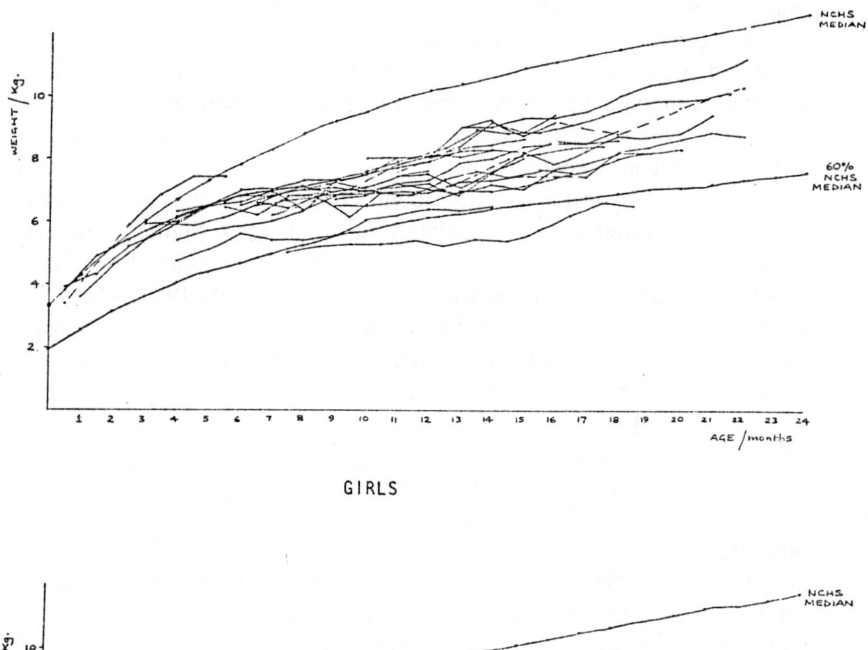

GIRLS

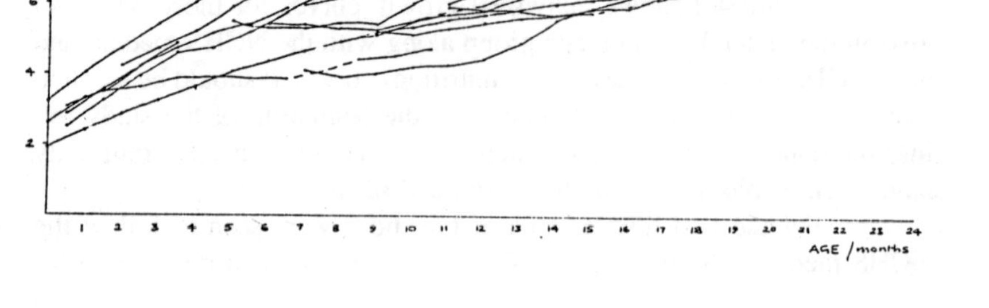

level off, and the biggest deviation from the median occurred between 6-12 months. After 12 months, the growth rate picked up again for several boys.

Girls generally appeared to have had lower birth weights than boys. They follow the NCHS median, but at a lower level than boys, until 4-6 months when growth rate decreased. After 6 months, there was no common pattern for girls, except that deviation from the NCHS median increased with age. There was much more inter-individual variation with girls than with boys, particularly up to 10 months.

4.2 SEASONALITY OF CHILD NUTRITIONAL STATUS

4.2.1 Overall Under-Fives

The overall monthly mean Z scores and percentage NCHS medians of the three anthropometric indices for all under-fives are graphed in Figure 4.2. Similar seasonal patterns were revealed with these two measures, but for later analyses where data were disaggregated by age and sex, Z scores were used, as their cut-offs take into account the variation of the coefficient of variation statistic with age, which percentage median cut-offs do not (Waterlow *et al.* 1977).

Examining Figure 4.3, it may be seen that the WH index was the most sensitive indicator in identifying seasonal changes in nutritional status. The range of seasonal change as measured by WH was greater and the coefficient of variation consistently smaller than the WA index.

Weight-for-height (WH) means remained roughly constant throughout summer. After the onset of the rains in June, they dropped to a low in August (86.7% median, -1.46 Z score). By October, however, the mean WH was back up to its summer level and later, in November, it reached its annual peak (90.3% median, -1.1 Z score) before tailing down slightly in December. Seasonally, the highest WH means were in winter; the lowest in the rains. The greatest monthly drop was in July; the greatest gains in September and October. The WA means showed a similar, though less marked, seasonal pattern.

The seasonal dimensions of malnutrition amongst under-fives with its rainy season peak were similar to findings of a number of studies reviewed by Schofield (1974), Longhurst and Payne (1979), and Chambers (1983), but contrary to the results of a recent South Indian study (Ryan *et al.* 1984).

FIGURE 4.3 : MONTHLY MEAN Z-SCORES AND PERCENTAGE NCHS MEDIAN OF THREE ANTHROPOMETRIC INDICES

LEGEND :
—— weight-for-age
- - - - height-for-age
•——• weight-for-height

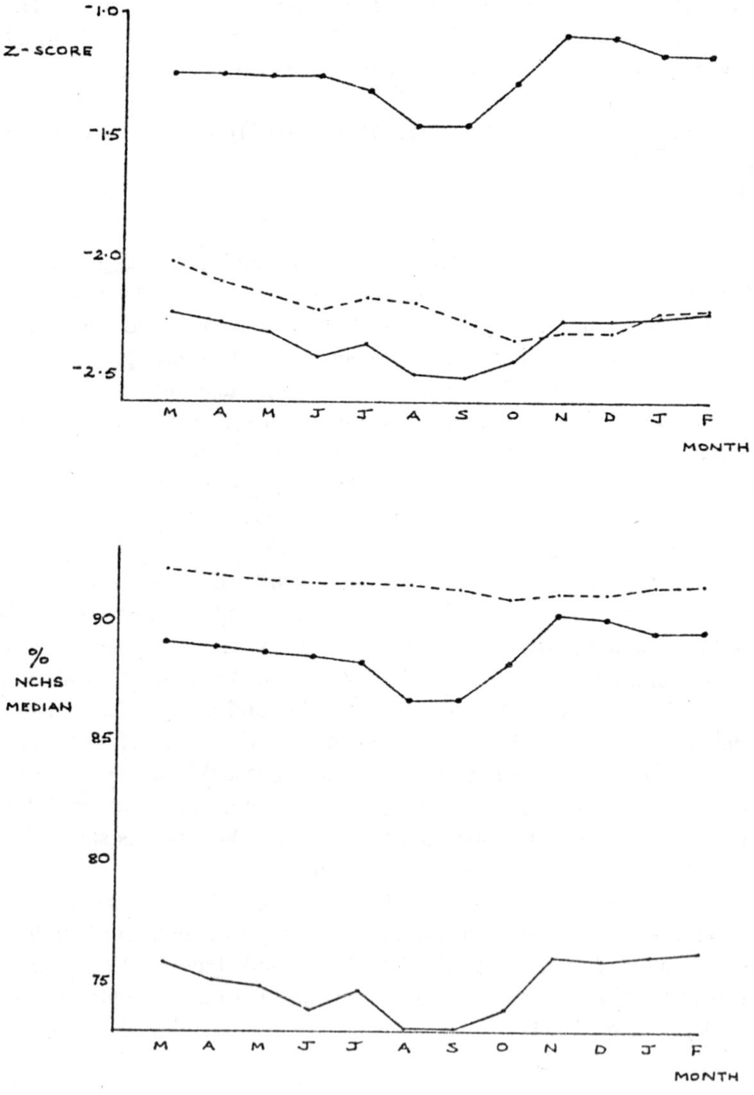

FIGURE 4.4 : AGE-SEX BREAKDOWN OF WEIGHT-FOR-AGE : MONTHLY MEAN Z-SCORES

LEGEND : —— BOYS ; - - - GIRLS

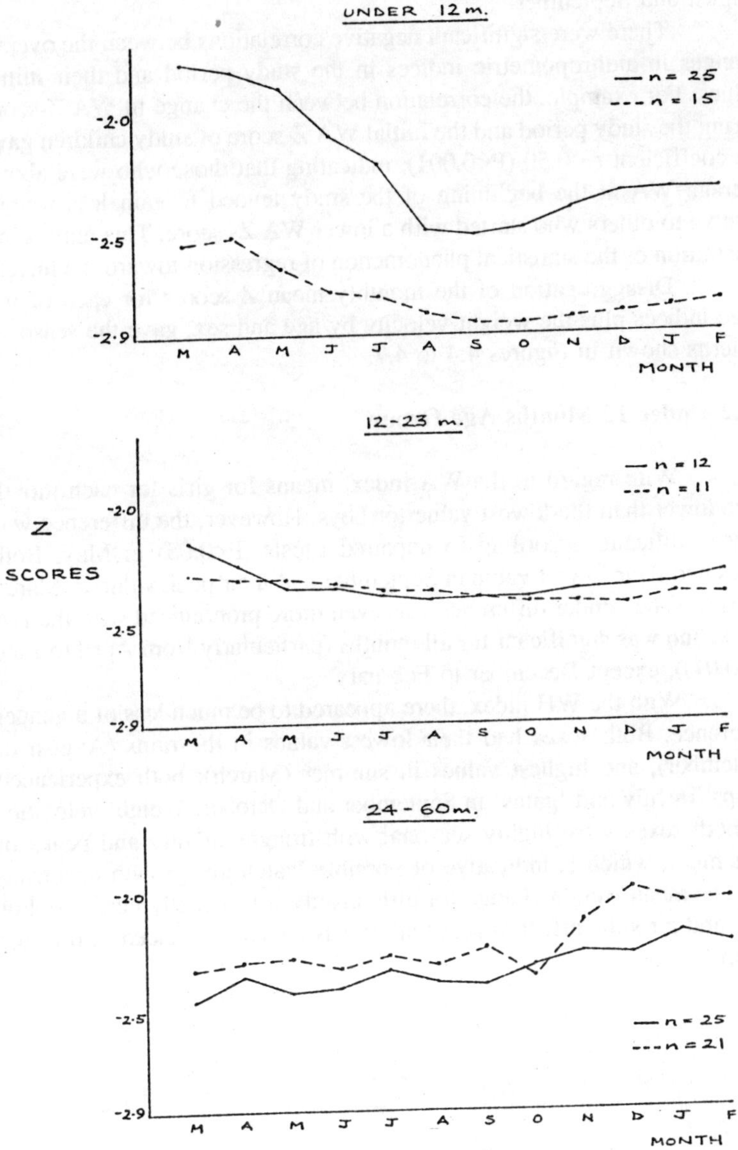

Least seasonal variation was apparent with the HA index. There appeared to be a lag behind the WH and WA indices, in terms of when the rainy season drop occurred, which is a common phenomenen (Brown *et al.* 1982; Chambers 1983). With the HA index, decreases occurred in August and September.

There were significant negative correlations between the overall changes in anthropometric indices in the study period and their initial values. For example, the correlation between the change in WA Z-score during the study period and the initial WA Z-score of study children gave the coefficient $r=-0.50$ ($P<0.001$), indicating that those who were above average WA at the beginning of the study tended to gain less weight relative to others who started with a lower WA Z- score. This may be an illustration of the statistical phenomenon of regression toward the mean.

Disaggregation of the monthly mean Z scores for each of the three indices plus the weight velocity by age and sex, gave the seasonal patterns shown in Figures 4.4 to 4.7.

4.2.2 Under 12 Months Age Group

With regard to the WA index, means for girls for each month were lower than the lowest value for boys. However, the difference was only significant, according to unpaired t-tests ($P<0.05$) in May. Both sexes had their lowest value in September and their peak value in March or April. The gender difference was even more pronounced with the HA index, and was significant for all months (particularly from April to June ($P<0.01$)), except December to February.

With the WH index, there appeared to be much less of a gender difference. Both sexes had their lowest values in the rains (August or September), and highest values in summer (March); both experienced 'drops' in July and 'gains' in September and October. Weight velocities for both sexes were highly seasonal with troughs in July and peaks in September, which is indicative of possible 'catch up' growth occurring (1). The mean weight change for girls in July was actually negative. For boys and girls the effect of seasonality was most pronounced in this age group.

FIGURE 4.5 : AGE-SEX BREAKDOWN OF HEIGHT-FOR-AGE :
MONTHLY MEAN Z-SCORES

LEGEND : ——BOYS ; - - - GIRLS

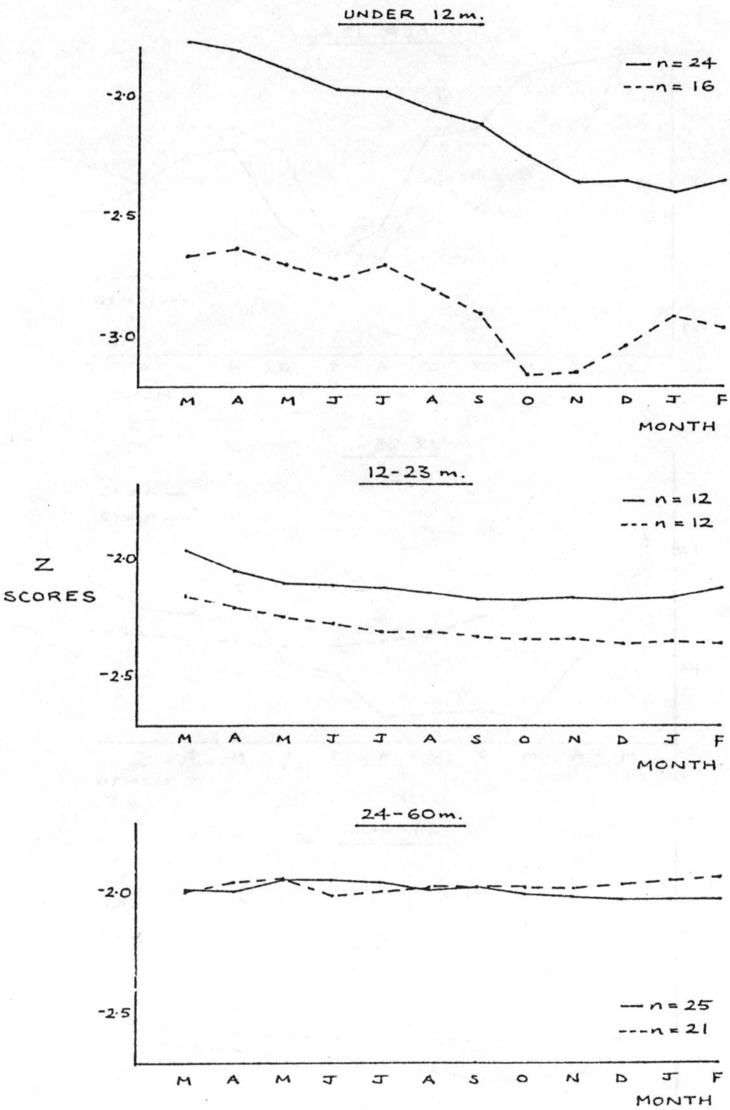

FIGURE 4.6 : AGE-SEX BREAKDOWN OF WEIGHT-FOR-HEIGHT : MONTHLY MEAN Z-SCORES

LEGEND : —— BOYS ; - - - GIRLS

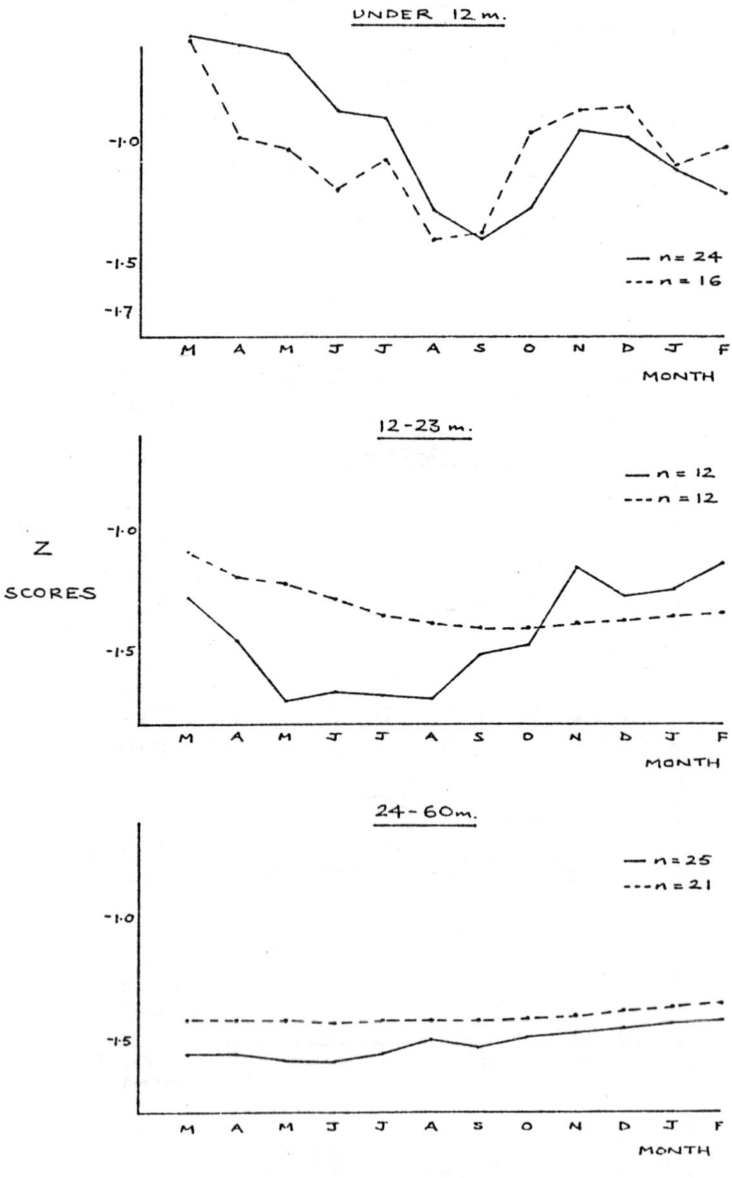

FIGURE 4.7 : AGE-SEX BREAKDOWN OF WEIGHT VELOCITY : MONTHLY MEAN WEIGHT GAIN

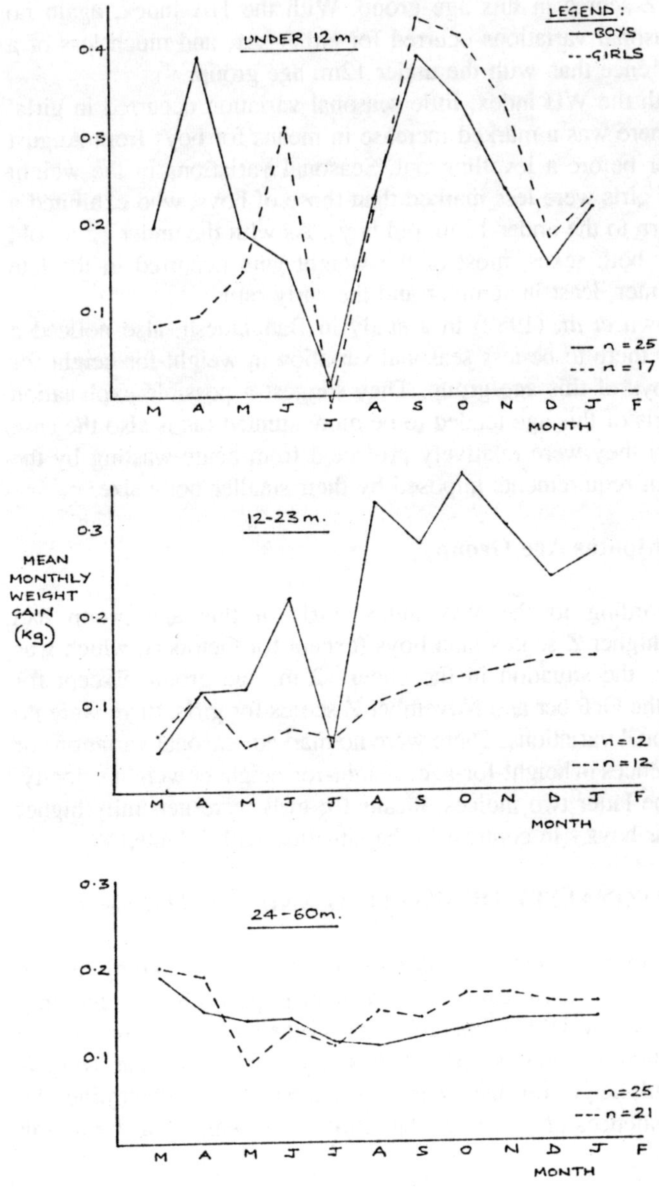

4.2.3 12-23 Months Age Group

There were no apparent seasonal variations or gender differences in the WA Z-scores in this age group. With the HA index, again no apparent seasonal variations ocurred for either sex, and much less of a gender difference than with the under 12m. age group.

With the WH index, little seasonal variation occurred in girls' means but there was a marked increase in means for boys from August to November before a levelling out. Seasonal variations in the weight velocities of girls were less marked than those of boys, who exhibited a similar pattern to the under 12 m. old boys. As with the under 12 m. old children, for both sexes, most of the weight gain occurred in the late rains and winter, least in summer and the early rains.

Brown *et al.* (1982) in a study in Bangladesh, also noticed a tendency for there to be less seasonal variation in weight-for-height for girls than boys of this age group. They suggest a possible explanation that since girls of this age tended to be more stunted (as is also the case in this study) they were relatively protected from acute wasting by the lower nutrient requirements imposed by their smaller body size.

4.2.4 24-60 Months Age Group

According to the WA index, girls in this age group had consistently higher Z scores than boys (except for October), which was in contrast to the situation in the under 12 m. age group. Except for increases in the October and November Z scores for girls, there were no marked seasonal variations. There were no marked seasonal variations or gender differences in height-for-age, weight-for-height or weight velocity, though for the latter two indices, means for girls were generally higher than those for boys - in contrast to the situation with infants.

4.3 SEASONALITY OF WASTING AND STUNTING

The monthly categorisation of under-fives according to the Waterlow Z score classification is shown in Figure 4.8. The monthly measurements for weight and height, expressed simply as greater or less than 2 standard deviations (SD) below the NCHS median weight-for-height and height-for-age, were cross-tabulated to determine the monthly prevalences of 'wasting', 'stunting' and 'wasting and stunting combined', as described in section 2.2.4.

Overall, approximately 50% suffered purely from stunting, and 3- 14% children, purely from wasting. The 'wasting and stunting combined' category contained from 6.9% (November) to 21.1% (June). Most wasting occurred in the summer and rainy season, and decreased fairly markedly after the rains in October, when stunting reached a high level. Throughout the whole year, however, about 30% children were defined as being 'normal', without wasting or stunting.

The sex-specific monthly prevalences are shown in Figure 4.9, and compared using Chi sq. analysis. The following points are made:

- The prevalence of pure stunting was over 50% throughout the year for girls; with boys, it was less than 40% for summer and the rains, before increasing to over 50% in winter. From March to May, and in October, these gender differences were very significant (P<0.01); less so in June and August (P<0.05), and non-significant in the other months.

- The prevalence of pure wasting fluctuated throughout the year for both boys and girls, ranging from 0% to 17.5% (boys) and 4.5% to 10.5% (girls). Gender differences were not significant except for February (P<0.01).

- The prevalence of wasting and stunting combined ranged from 8% (February) to 23.5% (April) for boys, and from 0% (March) to 23.1% (June) for girls. Boys had highest prevalences in the summer, least in the winter, while girls had highest prevalences in the rains, least in winter. These gender differences were very significant in March (P<0.01) and less so in April and July (P<0.05). Using Chi- squared analyses, (with the appropriate corrections for small expected frequencies where required), and cross-tabulating 'wasting and stunting combined' against the other categories combined, the seasonal variations in 'wasting and stunting' for girls, with its rainy season peak, emerged as being significant (Chi sq. = 21.0 11 d.f. P<0.05), while those for boys were not (Chi sq. = 11.3, 11 d.f. P>0.1).

The main gender differences thus were in the relative proportions of stunting and the seasonal variations in the proportions suffering both wasting and stunting. A higher proportion of girls suffered stunting than boys, and there was a marked seasonal variation in the percentage of girls with wasting and stunting combined, with the peak in the rainy season. A higher proportion of girls than boys were thus in the highest risk category at a time when, as will be shown in section 4.5, disease incidence was peaking.

FIGURES 4.8 and 4.9

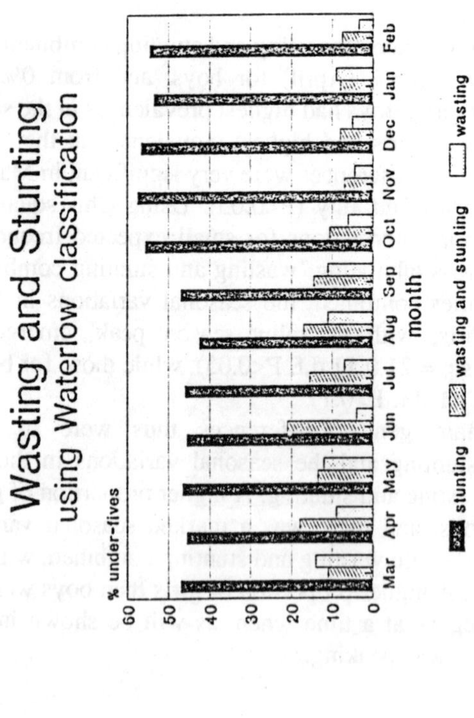

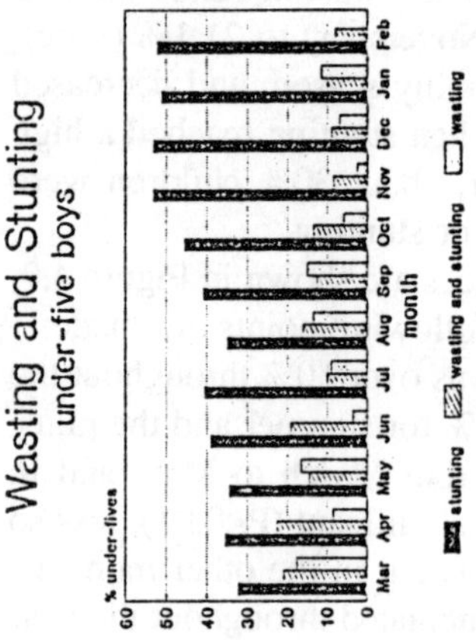

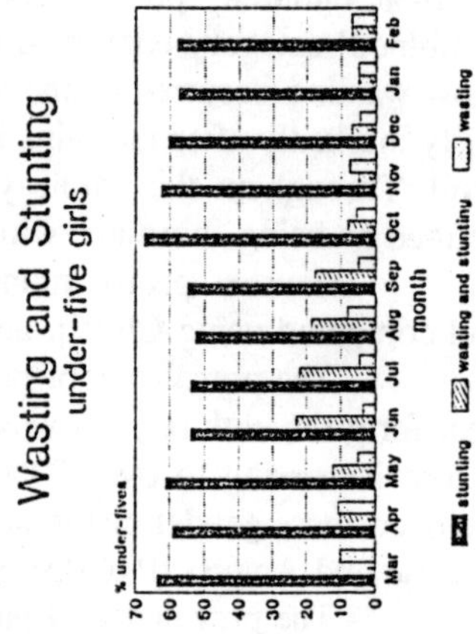

4.4 INTRA-HOUSEHOLD ANTHROPOMETRIC PATTERNS

The results of the classification discussed in section 2.2.3 were tabulated on a household-by-household basis and shown in Table 4.2. Those patterns suggested by Dugdale (1985) were found to be applicable, though with some modifications (in the case of patterns C and D), and additions (patterns G and H). Percentages of households that exhibited each pattern are shown in the table. Interpretations of the patterns are as follows :

Pattern A. The current nutrition of all family members is adequate. The parents and older children may be small in stature, reflecting chronic growth retardation in early childhood, but their present nutritional status is satisfactory.
Pattern B. The adults, infant and older children are all adequately nourished, but the 1 to 5 year old children show evidence of current growth retardation, possibly due to their no longer being protected by breast-feeding and their having difficulties in weaning.
Pattern C. There were three variants to this pattern, but in all households that exhibited it the mother and any elder children are adequately nourished unlike the youngest child. This suggests poor practices of infant and child care, perhaps of a working mother who cannot feed and care for her youngest child during the day. If the child is being weaned s/he may be experiencing difficulties adapting to the adult diet.
Pattern D. Poor nutrition and/or disease in the mother is likely to be a primary factor leading to secondary effects in the younger children. Elder children can fend for themselves.
Pattern E. Indicates an absolute lack of food for the family.
Pattern F. With isolated 'malnutrition' of an elder child is likely to have resulted from disease (e.g. parasites).
Pattern G. The youngest child is adequately nourished despite the mother being 'malnourished'. Child care and feeding practices are likely to be satisfactory, but the mother's energy intake may be deficient and her energy requirement for work unfulfilled.
Pattern H. The mother and youngest child are adequately nourished, while the father and possibly an elder child are 'malnourished'. Special attention may be being given to nutritionally vulnerable household members.

TABLE 4.2 : ANTHROPOMETRIC PATTERNS OF STUDY HOUSEHOLDS

PRESENT NUTRITIONAL STATUS OF.....

PATTERN	FATHER	MOTHER	INFANT	1-5 YR. OLD		>5 YRS. OLD			%
				1	2	1	2	3	
A	+	+	+	+	-	+	+	-	4.6
B	+	+	+	o	o	+	+	-	0.0
C1	+ or o	+	o	o	-	+	-	-	7.7
C2	+ or o	+	-	o	-	+	-	-	15.4
C3	o	+	-	o	o	+	-	-	12.3
D	+ or o	o	o	o	-	+	+	-	16.9
E	o	o	o	o	o	o	-	-	16.9
F	+	+	+	+	-	+	o	+	4.6
G	+	o	-	+	-	o	-	-	13.9
H	o	+	-	+	-	+	o	-	7.7

LEGEND : + weight-for-height satisfactory
o weight-for-height below cut-off
\- no family member
% percentage households

Overall, examining the relative percentages of households that exhibited each pattern, the main nutritional problems would seem to be those that relate to:

- Poor practices of infant and child care as a possible consequence of the mother's need to work, (35.4% households exhibited pattern C).
- Inadequate food entitlements at the household level (16.9% households exhibited pattern E).
- Adult female morbidity or 'malnutrition' repercussing on the infant, (16.9% households exhibited pattern D).

With regard to the 8 households with severely WA malnourished under-five children, 5 were in pattern E, 2 in D and 1 in C. Therefore, nearly half of all households (5 of 11) that exhibited patterns representative of aggregate household food shortage, contained an under-five year old child with severe malnutrition. Only 4 households did not contain any malnourished members.

Similar to the results of a study in Tamil Nadu by McNeill (1986), there was some evidence here of a wider extent of adult male than adult female malnutrition at the time of this whole household study in August. This type of gender difference has been postulated by Stini (1981) as being an effective adaptive mechanism which allows preservation of the child-bearing role of women.

Although the percentages of men and women in the middle two BMI categories were equal, there were relatively more men than women with BMIs less than 17.0 and twice as many women than men with BMIs greater than 20.0. The BMI distribution of women was skewed to the right of that of men. Chi-squared analysis, however, revealed the gender differences in the overall proportions to be non-significant (Chi sq. = 3.0; 3 d.f.; P>0.1).

These results, however, differed from the findings of the A.P. state-wide NNMB survey (1981), which gave mean BMIs (calculated from mean weights and heights) of 18-30 year old men and women of 18.8 and 18.1 respectively.

Eight patterns were identified here within the simplified framework adopted where analysis was confined to parents and their offspring. The diversity of patterns exhibited in the more complex reality of differing family types may in some societies defy meaningful classification. In order to maintain some degree of simplicity, and for the patterns to be useful in the particular context of the study hypothesis, it was felt necessary in some cases to make some value judgements in defining patterns. Hence patterns C and D were primarily defined according to the nutritional status of the mother and youngest child, while the father's nutritional status was variable. More in-depth work, e.g. case studies of households exhibiting a range of different patterns, would also be needed to determine how valid the interpretations of these patterns are in the particular social and environmental context.

TABLE 4.3 : ANTHROPOMETRIC MEASUREMENTS OF PARENTS

				BMI CATEGORY (% parents)			
	Wt(kg)	Ht(m)	BMI	<17.0	17.0-18.5	18.5-20.0	>20.0
Fathers	49.9	1.66	18.0	22.4	41.8	26.9	8.9
Mothers	43.2	1.52	18.7	13.4	41.8	26.9	17.8

4.5 SEASONALITY OF DISEASE INCIDENCE

4.5.1 Overall Under-Fives

The seasonal pattern of disease incidence in under-fives is illustrated in Figure 4.10. Diarrhoea was the most common childhood disease, as recalled by the mother. Its incidence followed a marked seasonal pattern, with a peak in July (34%), and a trough in November (10%). For each month in the rainy season, diarrhoeal disease incidence was above 20%, while in winter, monthly incidence was always below 15%.

Other common diseases recalled included skin and ear infections, colds, coughs and fever. There were two outbreaks of conjunctivitis (in July and September) in the study villages. Overall disease incidence was highest in July (52%), (followed by April and September (43%)) and lowest in the winter months (October to January), when it remained fairly constant at about 20%. There were dramatic drops from September to October in overall and diarrhoeal disease incidence. Monthly variations in overall disease incidence for all under-fives were shown by Chi-squared analysis to be highly significant (Chi sq. = 60.3, 10 d.f. P<0.001).

FIGURE 4.10 : SEASONALITY OF OVERALL (A) AND DIARRHOEAL (B) DISEASE INCIDENCE

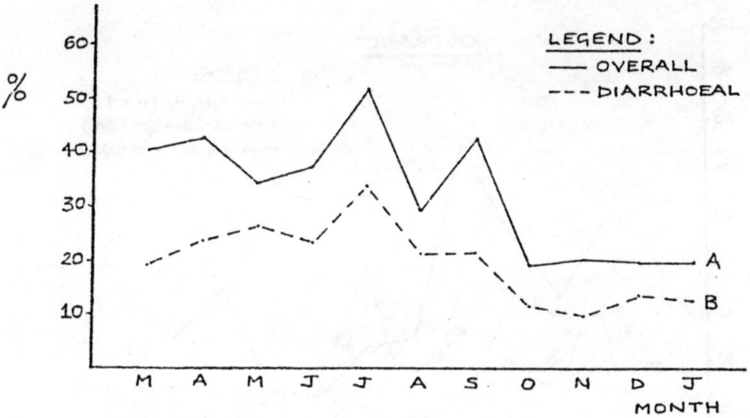

4.5.2 By Age and Sex

The age-disaggregated seasonal patterns of overall and diarrhoeal disease incidence are illustrated in Figure 4.11. Most seasonality was exhibited by the under 12 m. age group, with incidence ranging from 23% in October to 76% in July. The under 12 m. group also had the highest monthly levels of incidence, except in September and October, when the 12-23 m. group did. Chi-squared analyses revealed monthly variations in disease incidence to be highly significant for under 12 m. children, less so for 12-23 m. olds and insignificant for 24-60 m. olds (see Table 4.4).

Most seasonality in diarrhoeal disease incidence was observed in the < 12m. group (where peak incidence was 61% in July, as compared to a low of 8.5% in November), and least in the 24-60 m. age group (with a peak in August of 20%, and a low in January of 5.5%).

Overall, for under fives, there were no significant gender differences in either monthly overall or diarrhoeal disease incidence. A similar finding emerged from another study in Bangladesh (Chen and da Souza 1981), leading the authors to claim that preferential child care

FIGURE 4.11 : AGE BREAKDOWN OF OVERALL AND DIARRHOEAL DISEASE INCIDENCE

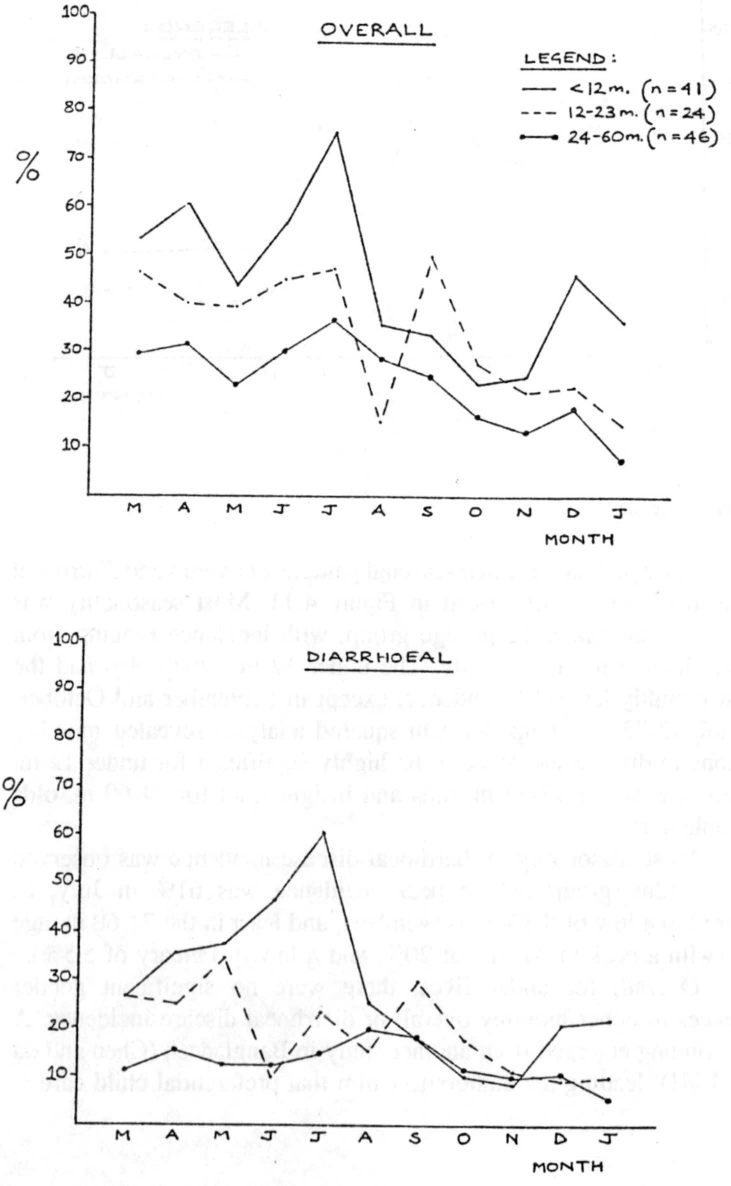

FIGURE 4.12 : AGE-SEX BREAKDOWN OF OVERALL DISEASE INCIDENCE

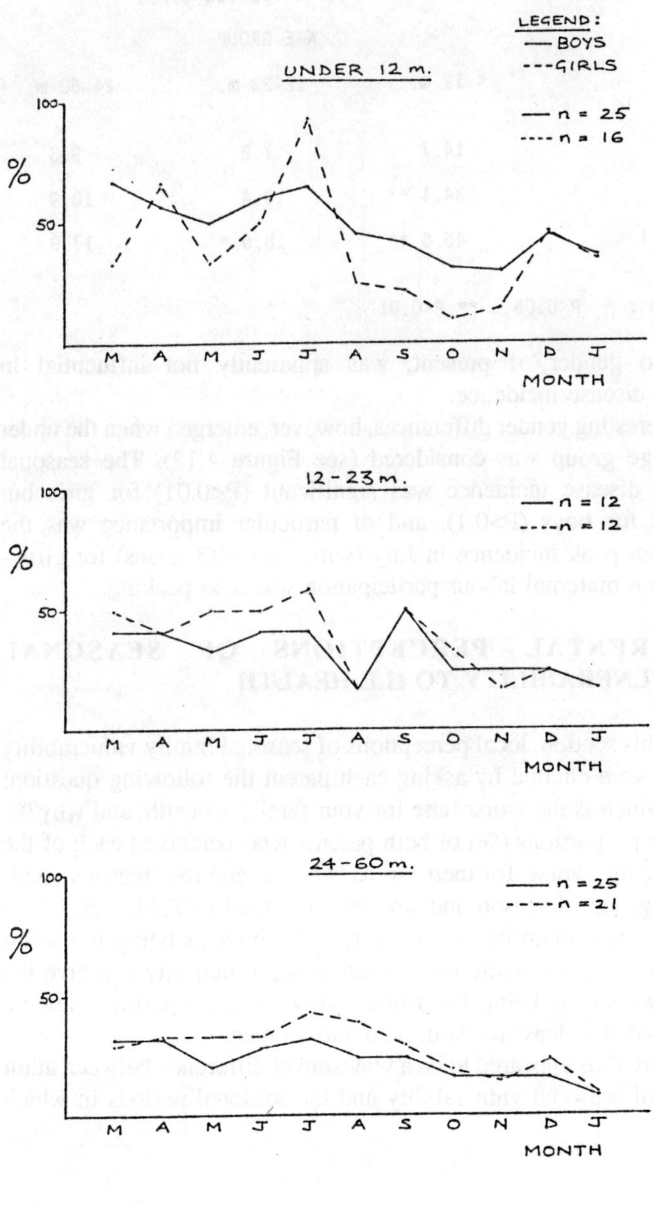

TABLE 4.4 : SEASONAL VARIATIONS IN DISEASE INCIDENCE, BY AGE AND SEX (CHI SQUARED TEST)

	Chi sq. value (10 d.f.)		
	AGE GROUP		
	< 12 m.	12-23 m.	24-60 m.
Boys	14.7	7.2	9.3
Girls	34.4 **	13.4	10.9
Overall	46.6 **	18.6 *	17.9

LEGEND : * P<0.05, ** P<0.01

according to gender, it present, was apparently not influential in determining disease incidence.

Interesting gender differences, however, emerged when the under 12 month age group was considered (see Figure 4.12). The seasonal variation in disease incidence was significant (P<0.01) for girls but insignificant for boys (P>0.1), and of particular importance was the highly distinct peak incidence in July (with over 90% cases) for girls - a month when maternal labour participation was also peaking.

4.6 PARENTAL PERCEPTIONS OF SEASONAL VULNERABILITY TO ILL-HEALTH

In this section, local perceptions of seasonal family vulnerability to ill-health were elicited by asking each parent the following question: "In a year, which is the worst time for your family's health, and why?".

The proportions (%) of both parents who perceived each of the seasons as being 'worst' for their family's health and the 'reasons cited' for each subgroup of season and sex, are presented in Table 4.5.

The great majority of men perceive winter as being the worst time for family health, while for women, a slight majority perceive the rains, over winter, as being the worst season. The proportion viewing summer as worst is least for both men and women.

There thus appeared to be a widespread difference between adult perceptions of seasonal vulnerability and the seasonal periods in which children generally experienced their lowest growth rates. This difference is particularly evident when comparing male perceptions with child growth data; less so with women. The possibility that 1985 was an abnormal year seasonally was not supported by villagers' answers when this question was posed in early 1986. The data on reasons cited, reveal interesting gender differences in perceptions, which may reflect different interpretations of the questions asked, or different conceptualisations of 'health'.

TABLE 4.5 : PARENTAL PERCEPTIONS OF "WORST SEASON" FOR FAMILY HEALTH

	SEASON					
	SUMMER		RAINS		WINTER	
	M	F	M	F	M	F
"Worst season ?" (% by sex)	11.9	22.4	23.9	41.8	64.2	35.8
Reasons cited (% by sex for each season)*						
Cash shortage	25.0	10.0	7.6			
Food shortage			25.3		31.0	43.2
Unemployment	37.5	20.0				
Adverse weather	37.5	40.0	37.1	11.8	59.0	38.0
Unavailable credit					18.0	
Water shortage	12.5	20.0				
Too much work			15.0	53.0		12.5
Child care time constraint				23.5		6.3
More disease		10.0	15.0	17.6		

* percentages may add up to more than 100% owing to some people citing two reasons for their choice.

For men, the question was often answered from an individual perspective. For example, 59% of men cited adverse weather as being the reason for their choice of winter as the worst time. This may have been due to the fact that they had to spend many nights out in the fields on raised platforms guarding the ripening rice crop from wild pigs, and, as a result, often caught coughs and colds and became fatigued.

For women, on the other hand, 'health' seemed to be more related to the survival of the family unit than to economic gain. Women were more responsible for provisioning and maintenance of the household unit. Over-work, too little time for child care, inadequate water supplies and lack of adequate sanitation were the most common reasons cited by women for family ill-health. 87% of the women who believed the rains to be the worst time, cited over-work and inadequate time for child care as the reasons. Most women who saw winter as the worst time, cited decreased food availability (probably pre-harvest in this case) as the reason.

The Concept of Quantity and Quality of Blood

In these tribal groups, there is a widespread identification of blood with strength, and 'no blood' ('raktum laydu') seems to be the nearest concept to that of malnutrition. Thinness in children is a widely recognised symptom of 'no blood', while the cause of this condition is seen as being due to inadequate consumption of food, not enough strength in the body, or just 'no blood' - it itself is seen as a cause. In the Tridosha theory of disease, blood is considered to be one of the 'dhatus' (i.e. a modification of the five elements ('bhutas') of the body, which must be kept within proper proportions, within certain limits for health (Kutumbaiah 1969).

Many men felt they were healthiest in the rainy season because they were mobile in the fields and, according to one man, "the good blood courses through the body". Blood was believed to go bad if it was allowed to stagnate through prolonged inactivity. In this way, the availability of work, as well as being seen as having an economic benefit, was generally felt also to lead directly to better health. The benefits to health of this mobility were believed to outweigh the problems caused by the recognised increase in diarrhoeal diseases and malaria, unless the latter became debilitating.

This view, however, did not seem to be as commonly held by

women, possibly because the rainy season tasks of transplanting and weeding did not involve the degree of mobility of ploughing. This belief may go some way towards explaining the lack of recognition among men of the initial rains being a bad time for family health.

4.7 SEASONALITY OF HOUSEHOLD HEALTH EXPENDITURE AND CHILD MORBIDITY

Overall for the study population, the highest mean monthly health expenditure per CU was in winter (Rs. 18.4); the lowest in the rains (Rs.14.8). This was in direct contrast to the seasonal differentials in child morbidity, where the highest levels of disease incidence were in the rainy season; the lowest in winter. Comparing income groups (see Table 3.8), G1 households were seen to maintain a level of about Rs.20-22 per CU throughout the year. For G2 households, the range was Rs. 13.4-17.8 per CU; for G3, Rs. 12.4-16.8 per CU. One-way analyses of variance and Scheffe tests revealed that G1 households spent significantly more on health for each season than G2 and G3 households and this expenditure was not subject to much seasonal variation, unlike the latter two groups.

Seasonality in health expenditure bore little relation to seasonality in child disease incidence. Expenditure on allopathic medicines depended on access to clinics and the availability of income and time. In the rainy season, roads leading out of the forest were generally impassable and clinics in the nearest town, Narsampet, inaccessible. The opportunity cost of foregoing one days' labour in the rains was particularly high. Furthermore, although much wage labour was carried out at this time, there were generally delays in payment and, consequently, little cash available (often until the maize harvest in September).

Child morbidity may thus have particularly serious consequences in the rains due to these factors preventing access to allopathic health care at a time when exposure to disease peaks and child care and feeding practices may be disrupted by the heavy maternal work load.

In contrast, after the paddy harvest in winter, cash and time were available and clinics accessible again. More trips were made to the nearest town, Narsampet, by the villagers usually primarily for reasons other than health, although medicines were often purchased. Similar findings have come from Madhya Pradesh (Howard 1978), where seasonal extremes severely reduced the accessibility of a rural hospital to the potential patient.

4.8 GENDER DIFFERENTIALS IN CHILD NUTRITIONAL AND HEALTH STATUS

The influence of gender on child nutritional and health status was particularly marked and warrants a deeper investigation. Seven of the eight severely malnourished (WA) children were girls. Girls suffered more from stunting. There were, however, no significant gender differences in the proportions of children with wasting, according to the weight-for-height index.

Gender differences in nutritional status of children may arise as a result of gender differences in factors such as these :

- incidence and duration of disease
- access to health care and treatment
- food allocation behaviour and individual dietary intake
- breastfeeding behaviour (frequency and duration of feeding)
- weaning practices (age weaned, weaning diet, degree of supplementation)
- quantity and quality of child care

Gender differences were not significant in overall disease incidence, although among girls under 12 months, disease incidence far exceeded that for boys in July - a month of peak female labour demand, when weight velocity was actually negative. This may have contributed to the relatively high prevalence of 'wasting and stunting combined' among girls at this time of the year.

As differentials were only marked in the under 12 month age group, breastfeeding behaviour, weaning practices and child care were potentially important contributory factors; gender differences in which were hard to detect. However, it was observed by the investigator during the course of the study, that mothers were generally more likely to forego agricultural labour to feed and care for a male, as opposed to female, infant, particularly during periods of intense maternal agricultural activity e.g. transplanting and harvesting.

Gender differences in access to health care were not directly investigated and health expenditure data was not disaggregated by sex in this study. It should, however, be borne in mind that in only 20% households, women were involved in decision-making in matters relating to health (see Table 3.10).

It must be remembered that studies such as this one are carried out with survivors who have resisted the stress of malnutrition and disease. Comparing sex ratios in different age bands of the study population (see Table 2.1), they were seen to be roughly even for children and adults, but masculinised for infants. Unfortunately, no gender-differentiated mortality data have been collected in this area (to the investigator's knowledge), and cell sizes in micro studies such as this one, are much too small for demographic research. It is not known whether the infant mortality rate for girls is higher than that for boys.

Gender differentials in mortality, if they exist, are likely to be related to gender differentials in child nutritional status, the latter having been shown to be related to mortality risk below a certain threshold (see section 1.2.2). The current debate on differential female mortality in South Asia has been summarised by Harriss (1987). Differentials in child mortality and nutritional status are hypothesised as being related to female economic and social status which may be influenced by both material and cultural factors (Clark 1987)

Material explanations relate to the economic undervaluation of women (Bardhan 1985). This, in turn, depends on female labour demand, participation and earnings, as well as the gender distribution of inheritance rights (that governs control of property) and the exchange value of the female at marriage (reflected in dowry costs). Household income differentials may have paradoxical effects. In poorer households, women (who are less dowered) may participate more in the wage labour markets and suffer less from the adverse effects of patrilinearity. However, resources being more scarce, the results of less discrimination may nonetheless be more fatal.

Cultural factors determine not only the gender division of waged tasks within which market mechanisms may operate (see section 1.4.1), but also systems of property ownership. (Das Gupta 1987).

In this study, material factors appear to have been less important. Despite the fact that female participation and female income were generally high, there were gender differences in child growth. The process of Hinduisation which is diffusing throughout tribal societies in South India, with the practice of dowry becoming increasingly widespread and the costs of the dowered increasing, may here be reflected in the relative neglect of the nutritional and health needs of girls vis-a-vis boys.

Note

1. Interestingly, during the months of greatest growth, some children's increments in weight and height approximated and slightly exceeded those of the NCHS reference population. Thus, if these children could have maintained their optimal performance throughout the year, there would have been little difference between the nutritional status of the two populations. Unfortunately, however, even during the best months of the year, the village children were not able to 'catch-up' from their accrued deficits.

5

REPRODUCTIVE CRISIS

In the preceding chapters, the processes of household production and reproduction have been described, along with a profile of the nutritional and health status of children - one outcome of these processes. In this chapter, the household-level socio-economic data and the individual-level data on child nutritional and health status, will be integrated.

Firstly, the relationship between household income levels and child nutritional and health status will be examined. Secondly, an analysis of the linear association between socio-economic factors and child nutritional status will be undertaken, and finally, a deeper seasonal analysis of the relationship between maternal labour participation, time allocation, and child nutritional status will be developed to investigate the central study hypothesis.

5.1 HOUSEHOLD INCOME AND CHILD NUTRITIONAL AND HEALTH STATUS

5.1.1 Income Differentials in Child Nutritional Status

There were no significant income-group differences (P>0.05) in the proportions of children within each category of growth retardation (see Table 5.1) for each indicator, as revealed by Chi- squared analyses (Chi squared values for WA, HA and WH, with 6 degrees of freedom were 5.0, 5.2 and 3.9 respectively). It is interesting to note, however, that four of the eight severely (WA) malnourished children came from the poorest income group, and none from the richest. With a larger sample size, a negative relationship between household income and the prevalence of severe child malnutrition might have emerged (see section 6.1).

Disaggregating by age of the child, no significant income-group differences (P>0.05) arose in the proportions of children from different age groups (under 24 months versus over 24 months) suffering second or third degree growth retardation (WA Chi-squared = 2.41, 2 d.f.).

FIGURE 5.1 : INCOME GROUP BREAKDOWN OF MONTHLY WEIGHT-FOR-HEIGHT (% median)

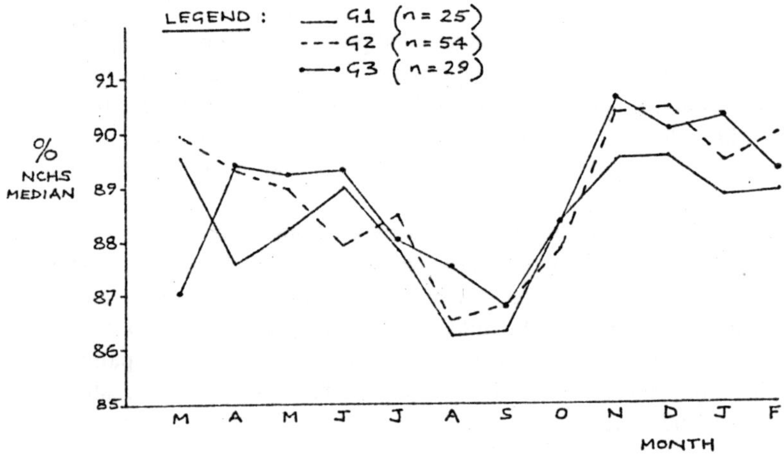

To investigate whether there were income differentials in the effect of seasonality on child nutritional status, the most sensitive seasonal indicator, weight-for-height, was selected and the data disaggregated by income group, giving the patterns shown in Figure 5.1. Each group exhibited a similar seasonal pattern, particularly after September. There were no significant income-group differences (P<0.05) in the WH means for each month, as detected by one-way analysis of variance.

Contrary to one of Chamber's major conclusions (1982), the children of less affluent households were not found to be more prone to seasonal malnutrition than those from richer households; a finding similar to that of Bairigi in a study in Bangladesh (1983). This again may have been due to the lack of marked economic inequality in this tribal community, where factors other than income come into play in explaining malnutrition.

5.1.2 Income Differentials in Child Morbidity

There were no significant income-group differences in the incidence of overall and diarrhoeal disease in any month (see Figure 5.2), as revealed by Chi squared analyses (i.e. Chi squared values were less than 5.99 (2 d.f.)). This concurred with results from a study in Sri Lanka (Watson 1984), but differed from the findings of a Bangladesh study (Becker *et al.* 1986) which showed that, despite the appearances of homogeneity of sub-optimal living conditions, socio- economic status variables were associated with differentials in child disease incidence. Income-group differences in this study were least in the rains and winter.

TABLE 5.1 : INCOME DIFFERENTIALS IN CHILD GROWTH RETARDATION (% children)

INDICATOR	INCOME GROUP	THIRD DEGREE	SECOND DEGREE	FIRST DEGREE	NORMAL
WA :	G1	0.0	46.1	53.9	0.0
(Gomez)	G2	7.1	44.6	48.3	0.0
	G3	13.3	30.0	56.7	0.0
HA :	G1	0.0	23.1	46.2	30.7
(Waterlow)	G2	7.1	25.0	53.6	14.3
	G3	10.0	20.0	50.0	20.0
WH :	G1	0.0	7.7	53.8	38.5
(Waterlow)	G2	0.0	10.7	53.6	35.7
	G3	0.0	13.3	33.3	53.4

Numbers (n) : G1 = 26, G2 = 56, G3 = 30

FIGURE 5.2 : INCOME GROUP BREAKDOWN OF OVERALL DISEASE INCIDENCE

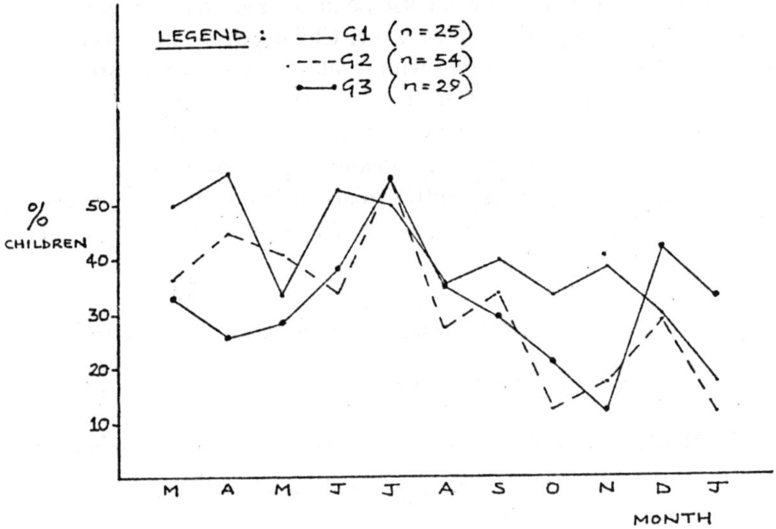

5.2 HOUSEHOLD SOCIO-ECONOMIC VARIABLES AND CHILD NUTRITIONAL STATUS

To examine possible linear trends in the association of the nutritional status of index children and demographic and socio- economic factors of their households, correlations of the mean annual WA Z-score of under-twos versus summary demographic and socio- economic variables were carried out.

Owing to the fact that severe malnutrition was only found in children under two years of age (who were anyway likely to be particularly dependent on the mother), only households with children of this age were considered in these analyses (n=65). In fact, there were only two households without under two year olds. The weight-for- age indicator was chosen as an indicator of nutritional status because, although it does not distinguish between current and long- term growth retardation, it is sensitive to both (1), and thus serves as a good single measure (Keller 1983). Correlation coefficients were determined, along with the level of their statistical significance (see Table 5.2).

TABLE 5.2 : CORRELATIONS OF MEAN ANNUAL WEIGHT-FOR-AGE Z-SCORE OF UNDER TWO YEAR OLDS VS. SUMMARY SOCIO-ECONOMIC VARIABLES

VARIABLE	CORRELATION COEFFICIENT (r)
Number of household members	0.01
Economic dependency ratio	0.09
Standardised operational landholding per CU	0.06
Total asset value per CU	0.10
Annual mean monthly maternal days worked	-0.32**
Annual mean monthly maternal wage days worked	-0.20
Total maternal income per CU	-0.11
Total paternal income per CU	0.01
Total cash income from agricultural labour per CU	-0.19
Total household income per CU	0.00
Months self-sufficiency in paddy	-0.08
Total loan taken per CU	-0.01
Mean monthly expenditure on staples per CU	0.07
Mean monthly expenditure on food per CU	0.16
Mean monthly expenditure on health per CU	-0.02
Mean daily household calorie consumption per CU	-0.09

LEGEND : * P<0.05, ** P<0.01

The only association that was statistically significant was that between maternal labour participation and child nutritional status. This is investigated in greater depth in the next section, where the effect of intervening factors is also taken into account.

5.3 MATERNAL LABOUR PARTICIPATION, TIME ALLOCATION AND CHILD NUTRITIONAL STATUS

5.3.1 Background

When a woman has the dual role of mother/housewife and labour force participant, trade-offs between child care and household maintenance and her extra-household labour activities may occur. Findings from a rural study in the Philippines indicated that the intra-household time substitutions, as a result of the mother's labour force participation, had net negative effects on the average nutritional status of children aged 1-71 months (Popkin 1980).

In contrast, Smith *et al.* (1983) found no relationship between the number of days the mother was away working and a decrease in her child's weight-for-age. Likewise, Ryan *et al.* (1984), and Blau (1981) did not detect a significant relationship between mother's hours of work and either child mortality or nutritional status.

Kumar (1978) in a study in Kerala, South India found that children whose mothers were in the wage labour force had significantly lower weights-for-age than children whose mothers did not engage in wage labour, even though per capita income was higher among families with mothers working. In families without mothers working, increases in family wage income had no incremental benefit on the children's nutritional status. Where mothers worked, their own wages had a positive effect on the nutritional status of their children. These somewhat conflicting results appear to have occurred because families with working mothers were generally poorer and their children more malnourished, but within that group mothers' incomes had a positive effect.

As described in the introductory chapter, the nutritional and health status of children are outcomes of household reproduction, which may be considered as being functions of the quantity and allocation of income and time. In this 'new home economics' approach, income may usefully be viewed as being related to food purchasing and production, and time as an important determinant of food production, preparation and feeding.

When the mother enters the labour force, the amount of time spent in work within the household (particularly more time intensive activities such as breastfeeding and child care), are likely to decline, while income and effective demand for food increase. Increases in female income may not, however, translate into increased energy intake of children, as child feeding is a time intensive activity, and the gender control of the disposition of this increased female income is obviously a critical factor. In a study conducted in villages of northern Ghana, Tripp (1981) found that the trading activities of the mother were the single most important determinant of the nutritional status of their children. Women traders controlled their earnings, which were used to purchase food.

Physical activity and social stimulation, as well as diet and health, may also affect the growth rate of children (Popkin and Solon 1976; Grantham-McGregor 1984). Time may affect other activities, including the mother (or surrogate) bringing the child for preventive health care such as immunizations, protecting the child from unsanitary conditions, and providing a clean and more healthy environment. Fuel and water collection, and food gathering may be constrained by lack of time available.

The educational level of the mother may be seen as enhancing the efficiency of combining income and time to produce adult and child nutrition. Inter-household differences in the level of maternal education, however, were negligible in the study area - the vast majority of mothers had not had any formal education.

The mother's dilemma between the need to maintain household food security through agricultural work and the need to adequately feed and care for her child may be at its most acute when the birth of a child coincides with a period of peak labour demand. This coincidence may lead to an increased risk of infant and child mortality (Crookes and Dyson 1981) and/or have an adverse effect on the efficacy of breast-feeding (Rajagopalan *et al.* 1981).

The net impact of maternal labour participation on child nutrition depends on intervening factors, other than household and maternal income. The type of labour and its compatability with child care and the quantity and quality of child care provided by the mother-substitute are of particular importance here.

5.3.2 Analysis

In order to investigate the seasonal association of maternal labour participation with child nutritional status, linear correlations were performed at three seasonal points corresponding to summer, rains and winter. With the time allocation variables, only the 24 households in the sub-sample were considered. The independent variables considered were:

- Mean monthly aggregate (wage and non-wage) days worked by the mother (hitherto 'maternal labour participation')
- Mean number of hours spent per day by the mother in child care (hitherto 'maternal child care')
- Mean number of hours spent per day by the mother and father in child care (hitherto 'parental child care')

The dependent variable was the weight-for-height Z-score. This indicator is a measure of wasting, or current nutritional status and has been seen to be the most sensitive to the effects of seasonality (see section 4.2). It was also found to have the strongest association with mean annual maternal labour participation ($r=-0.40$; $P<0.001$). As shown in section 5.2, weight-for-age also had a significant negative relationship ($r=-0.32$; $P<0.01$), unlike height- for-age ($r=-0.21$; $P>0.05$).

Weights-for-height of under twos were taken at the beginning of the months that marked the end of the season to which the labour participation variables applied (i.e. June, October and February). With regard to the time allocation data, weights-for-height of the under twos in the sub-sample were taken in April, August and December i.e. directly after the seasonal studies.

Maternal labour participation was significantly inversely associated with child nutritional status in the rains and winter, particularly the rains. The positive association with maternal and parental child care was only significant in the rains. There was a degree of collinearity[1] between the maternal and parental care variables, but it is interesting to note that the incorporation of time allocated to child care by the father, in the 'parental care' variable, effectively diluted the strength of association with child nutritional status - a rough indication of the superior quality of maternal child care.

The levels of significance of the latter correlations were not as great as those for maternal labour participation, which was not really surprising as only one day per season was measured and only 24 households were included in the time allocation studies.

TABLE 5.3 : SEASONAL CORRELATIONS OF MEAN WEIGHT-FOR-HEIGHT Z-SCORES OF UNDER TWOS WITH MATERNAL LABOUR PARTICIPATION AND TIME ALLOCATION DATA

VARIABLE	CORRELATION COEFFICIENT (r)
Summer :	
Maternal labour participation	-0.15
Maternal child care	0.24
Parental child care	0.20
Rains :	
Maternal labour participation	-0.46**
Maternal child care	0.46*
Parental child care	0.41*
Winter :	
Maternal labour participation	-0.30*
Maternal child care	0.38
Parental child care	0.34

LEGEND : * P<0.05, ** P<0.01

5.3.3 Effect of Household Income and Type of Labour

There was a negative (r = -0.20), but insignificant relationship between female wage-labour days worked and the WH Z-score of under two year olds. Households with high levels of maternal labour participation were not necessarily from poorer households. Women from richer households usually contributed much of their labour to own- farm production (see Table 3.4). Maternal labour participation was slightly negatively associated with total household income per CU (r = -0.21), but this was not significant. In the rainy season (a period of peak female labour demand) there was no relationship between maternal labour participation and income (r = -0.03). So it was the total number of days worked per month (whether waged or unwaged labour) which was significantly related to child nutritional status.

In contrast, Kumar (1978) found that a slow down in under 18 month old childrens' weight gain occurred only among children whose mothers were in the work force, but outside the home enterprise (i.e. the poorest, who relied on casual rather than self-employment), due to the different levels of compatability of waged and on-farm work with child care.

In this study area, however, compatability did not generally differ greatly between waged and on-farm labour, inasmuch as both types of work involved time-intensive activities (e.g. transplanting, weeding, harvesting), performed at some distance from the home. There were some differences though. Waged labour generally started earlier in the day than on-farm work, and on-farm workers were likely to have had more flexibility in terms of taking a break to feed an infant (which might have been brought to the mother in the field by an elder sibling).

5.3.4 Effect of Maternal Income

There was no relationship here between child nutritional status and the individual annual income earned by the mother. In fact, the individual maternal income was negatively correlated with child's weight-for-height Z-score (r = -0.11; P>0.05), as was the proportion of maternal to total agricultural labour income of the household (r=- 0.26; P<0.05). High female income households were among the poorest (see section 3.4.4), and it seems that the effect of this household- level poverty overrode the potentially beneficial effect of high female income on household calorie consumption and child nutrition. Maternal income, unlike total household income, was not positively correlated with mean daily household calorie consumption (r = -0.15). Furthermore, as shown in Table 3.10 women in general had little control over decisions regarding the disposition of income and expenditure on food.

5.3.5 Child Care by Mother-substitutes

Individuals assigned the task of looking after infants and young children were generally elder siblings or grandparents. Examples of the provisions made by mothers for the care of their children while they worked outside the household are detailed in section 6.3.

Each of the mothers of the other six severely malnourished girls participated in paddy transplanting in the child's first year of life. The examples cited below illustrate the particular constraints on child care and feeding at this time and the common inadequacies of child care by mother-substitutes:

One mother left her 9 month old child for 6 weeks to join a transplanting gang in a more remote village. Three of the girls (who were cousins) were left in the care of their grandfather, when their mothers were transplanting, though the latter endeavoured to return at midday to breastfeed them. One girl who weighed only 4 kg. at 7 months of age, was left, at 3.5 months, in the care of an elder sister during the day for the month of paddy transplanting. The sister would usually bring her to her mother in the field for midday feeding, but she was often asleep, and consequently not fed, when her mother returned at dusk.

5.3.6 Seasonality of Conceptions and Births

At this point it is useful to examine the seasonal trends in conceptions and births. The tendency for the birth rate in these villages to peak in the rainy season is illustrated in Figure 5.3. 49% of study children were born between June and September, with a peak in July. This corroborates evidence, cited earlier, that births tend to coincide with periods of increased female labour demand.

This July peak implies a peak in conception in October, when there is a slack period in agricultural labour demand, the weather is becoming cooler and the Dussera festival is celebrated. Studies in rural Bangladesh have also indicated that conception peaks during the cool season (Chen *et al.* 1974), and maybe related to increased coital frequency at periods of relatively low labour demand, when the husband is still at home and has not temporarily migrated in search of work, as in summer (Shaikh and Becker 1985). If the peak female labour demand in July results in children being abruptly weaned off the breast, then, many women may resume ovulation in August/September, leading to the peak in conceptions observed in October.

Figure 5.3

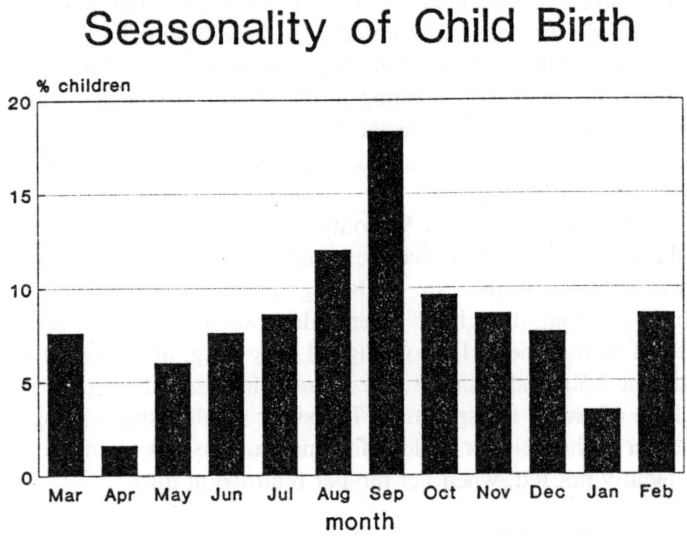

Whatever the mechanism responsible, however, the effect of child births occurring at such times is likely to be one of an increased risk of infant and child mortality. If the mother goes out to work, the efficacy of breast-feeding and child care is likely to be reduced, resulting in higher risks of the child becoming ill and/or malnourished. If she cares for the child at home, she forgoes earning, at a time when female income peaks, with possible adverse consequences for household food security.

As Schofield (1974) has shown, the issue of seasonal timing of conception to avoid birth during the rains is not simple. For example, babies born during the rainy season may be immediately vulnerable, but those born during the dry season become vulnerable later, when they lose passive immunity after 6 months during the following rainy season.

5.4 SUMMARY

The net effect of maternal labour participation and time allocated to activities incompatible with child care appeared here to have been detrimental to young dependent children. This relationship was found to be independent of household income (particularly in the rains when the effect was most marked) because virtually all women worked, and there were no significant income-group differences in the levels of aggregate maternal labour participation. Furthermore, although the ratio of waged to unwaged work did vary between income groups, the net effect of the compatibility of the work with child care and/or the adequacy of mother-substitutes appeared not to significantly differ for waged or unwaged workers.

The adverse effect of high maternal labour participation on child nutritional status is likely to have been predominantly due to both quantitative and qualitative effects on child care and feeding. Infants tended to be 'opportunity-fed' (as opposed to 'demand-fed'), a term used first by Bailey (1965) to describe the pattern of breastfeeding whenever the mother has a chance. These effects were particularly serious in the early rains, when high female labour demand and participation (e.g. paddy transplanting in July) coincided with high disease incidence amongst under-fives (particularly infants). At this time, child nutritional status was generally particularly low.

High levels of maternal income did not translate into improved child nutritional status as these households were among the poorest anyway, with low levels of food availability and consumption, and women generally had little individual control over the disposal of their income.

Correlation analysis reveals the degree of association between variables, but does not prove causation. In the following chapter, quantitative and qualitative data is used to reveal the network of relationships between different causal influences that exists in households with a severely malnourished child.

Notes

1. The correlation coefficients for the correlations of the annual mean values of the three anthropometric indices for all the study children revealed this. They were :

   Weight-for-height vs. height-for-age (r=0.24)
   Weight-for-age vs. height-for-age (r=0.81)
   Weight-for-age vs. weight-for-height (r=0.69)

6

THE SEVERELY MALNOURISHED

In this chapter, in order to gain a deeper understanding of the interaction of the determinants and processes that result in severe malnutrition, a characterisation of households with severely malnourished children will be carried out. Detailed profiles of two families are also presented to illustrate the nature and quality of the mother-child relationship and the social and economic constraints that operate on it.

6.1 DISTINGUISHING FEATURES OF 'SEVERELY MALNOURISHED HOUSEHOLDS'

In order to reveal characteristics of households with severely malnourished children, the study households were initially divided into two groups - those households with a severely malnourished child (hitherto referred to as 'severely malnourished households' for short), and those without severe malnutrition. The weight-for-age indicator was employed owing to its high discriminatory power with respect to mortality risk (see section 1.2.2), and the fact that it is a good composite measure of both long-term and recent growth retardation (see section 5.2).

Again, as severity of malnutrition has been shown to vary with age, the age group of the index child used to classify the household has to be specified (1). Only those households which contained children from the age groups which contained severely malnourished children will be considered in this particular analysis. The two groups of households were:

i) households containing children whose mean annual weight-for-age (WA) was less than 60% NCHS median, i.e. fell into the 'severe' category of the Gomez classification (n=8).

ii) households containing children from the same age group, whose mean annual WA was greater than 60% NCHS median (n=57).

A second type of categorisation was carried out to determine whether there were features common to households with severe child malnutrition, apart from poverty or malnutrition, which distinguished them from other households. The above categorisation was thus standardised with respect to household income, giving the following groups:

i) households with 'severe' malnutrition, as defined above (n=8)

ii) households without 'severe' malnutrition up to the income ceiling (total household income per CU) of the richest 'severely malnourished household' (n=37).

For each of the above categorisations, the statistical significance of differences in means between subsamples, for summary socio-economic, demographic and individual variables, was determined by employing Student's unpaired t-test, which has been shown to be 'robust' in non-extreme departures from normality of data (Kirkwood 1988).

The characteristics outlined below were those that distinguished the severely malnourished subsample from the other subsample in each respective categorisation. Owing to the small cell sizes, a two-tailed probability value P<0.1, indicating at most a 1 in 10 chance of the null hypothesis being incorrectly rejected was taken as a cut-off to indicate 'significant' characteristics. With a larger sample size, some of these differences might have shown a higher level of significance. The t and P values for the tests with 63 (n-2) degrees of freedom are shown in parentheses.

6.1.1 Characteristics of 'Severely Malnourished Households'

Individual

- high annual mean number of disease episodes (t=2.1; P=0.04)

Socio-economic

- low standardised operational landholding size per CU (t=2.21; P=0.03)
- high annual mean monthly total days worked by mother (t=1.99; P=0.05)
- low total asset value per CU (t=1.85; P=0.06)

- low mean monthly cash expenditure per CU on health (t=1.73; P=0.09)

6.1.2 Characteristics of Income-standardised 'Severely Malnourished Households'

Individual
- high annual mean number of disease episodes (t=1.76; P=0.08)

Socio-economic
- no significant variable.

Child disease incidence was one of the most significant factors associated with child malnutrition, and was the only variable that remained as significant when the income ceiling was applied. This corroborates evidence cited by Tomkins (1985) that, as well as increased severity and duration of disease, severely malnourished children may have higher rates of disease incidence. Furthermore, this relationship was relatively independent of household income - a similar finding to those of studies by Watson (1984) and Victora *et al.* (1986).

Other characteristics of severely malnourished households included a high level of maternal labour participation and low values of variables that reflect household socio-economic status e.g. landholding size, total asset value, and health expenditure. Low household income per CU, however, was not quite a significant characteristic itself (P=0.12). Again, this may be partially due to the small cell size of the 'severely malnourished' group - with a larger sub-sample, significance might have emerged. This is investigated further in sections 6.2 and 6.3 below.

Low levels of household energy consumption per CU were not significant characteristics of these households either (P=0.15), though this was not really surprising, as most of the severely malnourished children were not yet solely dependent on the adult diet, and many were still being breastfed. Furthermore, no account of intra-household food allocation behaviour is incorporated in this aggregate variable. Maternal time allocated to child care and feeding is likely to have been a more significant nutritional factor than aggregate levels of household energy consumption for these children, especially given the co-incidence of high levels of both maternal labour participation and child disease incidence in the rains. There is a further disturbing co-incidence of high disease incidence in the index children with low levels of household health expenditure.

Due to the limited size of the time allocation study subsample, it was not possible to incorporate the child care time variables within the above analysis. However, maternal time allocation in the 'severely malnourished households' has been investigated in section 5.3.2 and the family profiles below. These present evidence for the existence of direct maternal time constraints in child care and feeding in these households.

6.2 CASE STUDIES

Summary demographic and economic characteristics of households with severely malnourished children are given in Table 6.1, while Table 6.2 shows details of the nutritional status of these children and their parents.

Table 6.1 shows that five of the eight households were Koya, four of which were from Musmi village. Family size and economic dependency ratio varied considerably between households - severe malnutrition was not concentrated in large families with high dependency ratios.

All households, except case 7 had landholdings per CU and total income per CU below the overall mean. Four households were in the poorest income group 3 (with one borderline G2/3), four in group 2, and none from the richest group 1. Both the absolute and relative levels of indebtedness varied widely between households. Mean monthly expenditure on health per CU for every household with severe malnutrition was below the overall mean. Both aggregate and waged maternal labour participation was higher than the overall mean in all but one household.

Only three households were defined as 'ultra poor', spending more than 80% total income on food, yet fulfilling less than 80 % household calorie requirements. So, contrary to Lipton (1983), household 'ultra poverty' in this study community was not closely associated with the risk of severe child malnutrition. This is probably related to the fact that consumption loans were not accounted for in the income variable, though they were used to purchase food.

Table 6.2 shows the highly pronounced gender differentiation of severe malnutrition, with only one boy and seven girls in this category. Ages varied from 0 to 20 months (at the beginning of the study) with a mean of 9.8 months. Six of the eight children were born in the rainy

TABLE 6.1 : DEMOGRAPHIC AND ECONOMIC CHARACTERISTICS OF 'SEVERELY MALNOURISHED HOUSEHOLDS'

	HOUSEHOLD NUMBER							
VARIABLE	1	2	3	4	5	6	7	8
Tribe	Koya	Koya	Koya	Koya	Lam.	Lam.	Koya	Lam.
Village	Mus.	Mus.	Mus.	Mus.	Than.	Rav.	Rav.	Rav.
Household members	6	5	7	6	4	9	7	3
Economic dependency ratio	0.55	0.49	0.25	0.60	0.42	0.58	0.60	0.21
Standardised land-holding per CU (ac.)	0.49	0.50	0.74	0.58	0.61	0.42	0.88	0.00
Total income per CU (Rs.)	991	1205	1552	1358	929	1123	1680	694
Income group	3	2	2	2	3	3	2	3
'Ultra poor' ?	-	Y	-	-	-	Y	-	Y
Energy consumption (kcals. per CU)	2320	2180	2330	2190	1960	1990	2770	1820
Food expenditure/ total income (%)	101	85	40	61	70	108	65	99
Total loan per CU (Rs)	246	189	80	501	1058	223	683	526
Total loan/income (%)	25	16	52	37	114	20	41	76
Monthly health expenditure per CU (Rs)	11.6	13.0	9.0	12.8	13.8	12.6	12.2	8.8
Aggregate maternal labour particip. (d)	16.4	17.3	14.1	16.5	15.9	16.7	17.4	18.0
Maternal wage labour participation (d)	8.3	9.6	3.2	7.9	8.4	10.1	9.0	18.0

TABLE 6.2 : NUTRITIONAL CHARACTERISTICS OF SEVERELY MALNOURISHED CHILDREN AND THEIR PARENTS

VARIABLE	HOUSEHOLD NUMBER							
	1	2	3	4	5	6	7	8
Index child								
Sex	F	F	F	F	M	F	F	F
Age in March 1985 (m)	9	19	11	6	8	0	20	6
Birth month	Jun	Aug	Apr	Sep	Jul	Mar	Jul	Sep
Annual mean :								
% WA	57.8	59.8	59.6	59.8	54.1	59.9	56.4	52.1
% HA	87.1	85.3	85.5	- *	85.1	85.7	85.1	84.1
% WH	77.2	77.6	81.0	- *	76.3	89.8	73.3	79.2
Months 'severe WA'	11	5	8	9	12	7	11	11
Morbidity (months ill)	5	5	3	4	6	4	4	6
(main season)	summ.	summ. wint.	summ. rains	summ. rains	rains	rains wint.	rains	summ. rains
Mother**								
Weight (kg)	42.0	40.9	38.3	47.2	38.1	39.2	37.0	36.0
Height (m)	1.55	1.47	1.49	1.61	1.47	1.46	1.48	1.44
BMI	17.5	18.9	17.2	18.2	17.6	18.4	16.9	17.4
Father**								
Weight (kg)	44.0	42.8	47.9	42.0	42.5	49.7	46.5	44.5
Height (m)	1.56	1.54	1.60	1.60	1.67	1.67	1.64	1.59
BMI	18.1	18.0	18.7	16.8	15.2	17.8	17.3	17.6
Household Pattern	E	C	D	E	E	E	D	E

* height measurements of the child in household 4 could not be taken as she had a deformed foot and the parents would not allow it.

** measurements taken in August.

season - a period of peak agricultural work load and generally high levels of morbidity among children (the implications of this were discussed in section 5.3.6). The number of months during which these children contracted illnesses varied from 3 to 6, with the rains, followed by summer being the main seasons.

The growth curves of these severely malnourished children were not smooth, indicating periodic growth checks, possibly as a result of regular bouts of illness. Only one child was in the 'severe' category for less than 6 months of the year, while four children were so classified in 11 or 12 months of the year.

Six mothers and seven fathers had BMIs below the cut-off of 18.5, of which one mother and two fathers had BMIs below the cut-off of 17. In five of the eight households with severe child malnutrition, all the other household members were classified as being 'malnourished' - a pattern indicative of an aggregate food shortage at the household-level. Other anthropometric patterns that emerged eluded to problems of child care and disease management (of the child and/or mother).

6.3 FAMILY PROFILES

In-depth qualitative and quantitative information on the following two households was collected by a combination of semi-structured interviews and participant observation throughout the year. The two households profiled were numbers 5 and 7 - the richest 'severely malnourished household' (from G2) and the poorest landed household with severe child malnutrition (from G3).

The profiles are structured in the following way. Firstly, the demographic composition of the household is outlined, followed by a description of its socio-economic status and food provisioning strategy. Secondly, the variations in nutritional and health status of the index child throughout the year are described. The nutritional and health status of the mother and the patterns of her labour participation and time allocation are then detailed, before a summary of the factors that appear to be related to the existence of severe child malnutrition in the household.

6.3.1 Family Profile 1

Household head:	Esam Palagaya
Tribe:	Koya
Village:	Ravenniguddem

Esam Palagaya (26) and his wife, Adama (25) had four daughters - Saroppa (7), Bartoma (5), Chamala (4) and Bagyama (20 months) - and one son, Giribabu (4 months). Palagaya has lived in the Musmi area since birth, while Adama lived in a Koya village in Badrachalam (about 50 km. away) until she married in 1977.

This household was the richest of those with severe malnutrition. It ranked at number 22 out of the 67 households in order of decreasing income per CU. Palagaya, an only son, inherited 3 acres of wet land and 1 acre of dry, when he married, for which he owns land deeds. With five children below the age of 7 years, however, the household economic dependency ratio was high.

He took two loans in 1985 - one of Rs. 1600 from a bank in Gudur, and one of Rs. 1500 from a private moneylender in Edelapelli - mainly for agricultural inputs, such as fertiliser, pesticide and any labour costs. Palagaya claimed the crop produce of his land was generally sufficient to feed the family for 9 months. Daily calorie consumption of 2770 kcals. per CU was the highest of any of the 'severely malnourished households' (see Table 6.1).

Bagyama was the fourth daughter, born July 1983, and the only child in the study population who was severely WH malnourished, as well as severely WA and borderline HA. Her growth curve was particularly striking and showed her to have been in the severe category for every month. Her weight-for-age increased gradually during April and May, dropped slightly in June with the onset of the rains, before plummeting in July and August (6.8 to 5.9 kg.). A period of 'catch up' growth then ensued with her gaining weight progressively from September to January, when she reached her peak WA of 60.6%

Bagyama had four bouts of illness during the study period - all during the rainy season. During June she suffered from acute conjunctivitis for nearly a week; in July she had diarrhoea and a fever for 10 days; in August, an ear infection also accompanied by a fever lasted for nearly two weeks, while, during September, she came down with a bad cold for 5 days.

Her brother, Giribabu, was born in December 1984, virtually blind, with his eyes only half-formed, possibly as a result of parental venereal disease. From birth, his WA (annual mean 64.9%) decreased steadily. Adama took him to the large government hospital in Warangal on several occasions in summer for tests. Adama herself was ill during the rains, contracting malaria in June. She spent the week prior to the onset of the rains in Polarem, a village 10 km. away, which was the home of a reputed local healer. Here she stayed for 5 days, sleeping in the open, beneath a tamarind tree, believed to be the home of a 'curing spirit'. During this time, the healer dispensed 'chettlu mandullu' and performed mantras daily, for a total cost of Rs. 50. Meanwhile, Bagyama, who had conjunctivitis, was being looked after by Palagaya. Adama returned in mid-June and went straight into agricultural work. When she was measured in August, her weight was just 37 Kg., and her BMI, 16.9. Despite her malnutrition she endeavoured to continue agricultural work, such as sowing, transplanting and weeding during the rainy season.

Adama divided her time between agricultural labour, whether waged or unwaged, and her domestic responsibilities. Preferential care was given to Giribabu, the only son, and Bagyama, the fourth daughter, who was just two years of age in July, was relatively neglected. She contracted diarrhoea with fever, and started to lose her appetite, refusing food. Her elder sisters, who were left at home to care for her and Giribabu, were content to leave her in the hut for most of the day. Saroppa regularly took Giribabu to Adama in the fields at midday for breast-feeding.

In August, Adama began to recognise Bagyama's increasingly critical condition, and she took her to the Polarem healer, who gave her a 'lekka borra' - a talismanic necklace with magical powers (consisting of a piece of tree bark and a piece of paper with a mantra inscribed by the healer, wrapped in a ball of thread).

Adama's family labour participation in the rains was particularly high as she carried out exchange labour for her father- in-law. She also hired herself out for agricultural labour. In October, her workload dropped considerably and she spent more time at home with Giribabu and Bagyama. Bagyama's health picked up, and she started to put on weight quite dramatically from September to December.

Severe malnutrition appears to have occurred in this household as result of a combination of factors e.g. high birth order and economic dependency ratio, regular infection of the child, high levels of maternal labour participation and maternal ill-health. Sibling sequence seems also to have had an adverse effect for Bagyama, the fourth daughter, born 16 months before the first son.

6.3.2 Family Profile 2

Household head: Wancrort Bikya
Tribe: Lambadi
Village: Musmi Thanda

Wancrort Bikya (20) and his wife, Jamu (19), had one son Ramesh (8 months). They lived with Bikya's widowed mother, Umballi. Bikya was the youngest of his father's three sons, and when he died, his land was divided between the three of them, and Bikya remained in the parental home with his mother after his marriage in 1983.

The family was one of the poorest in the study population (ranking 64 out of 67 in order of decreasing income per CU). Bikya had 0.75 acre of rainfed paddy and 2.5 acres of forest-cleared infertile land, for which he owned no land deeds. Consequently, he was ineligible for a loan from institutional sources, which probably accounted considerably for his position of extreme indebtedness. In 1985, he took out three loans from local private moneylenders, totalling Rs. 3300. The breakdown of the use for which these loan were intended was as follows : Rs. 1000 for agricultural inputs; Rs. 1000 for rice, pulses, cooking oil and health contingencies; Rs. 500 for spices and vegetables; Rs. 500 for new clothes.

His own crop produce, he claims, lasts for just 3 months. The daily household calorie consumption per CU from staple foods was very low (1960 kcals. per CU), at least partially due to the foregoing of a midday meal during peak workload periods in the rains and at harvest time. The household, however, was not classified as being 'ultra poor' on account of their having spent only 70 % of their income on food. However, as shown, consumption loans which are not included within the income variable were used for much of the food expenditure.

Bikya claimed that, despite the apparent cutting-back on household food consumption at certain times, he would always take a consumption loan "rather than starve. If we don't eat, our strength decreases, we can do less 'kuli' (wage labour), we become more ill and would have to spend more on medicine". The foregoing of the midday meal, when it occurred may have been as much a time constraint as an economic one - an illustration of the importance of these two factors in household nutrition.

Ramesh (born July 1984) had the lowest, but one, annual mean WA (54.1%), as well as having been borderline (severe/moderate) HA. Jamu claimed he was very small at birth. His growth curve remained below the 60% WA line for each month of the year. In the 7 months between March and September, Ramesh gained only 400g (from 5.0 to 5.4 kg.), before, at 15 months of age, he started to gain weight more rapidly between October and December.

Ramesh suffered regular bouts of illness in the summer and rainy season, particularly diarrhoea, often accompanied by fever. For most of the summer, he had scabies, and during the rains, he suffered from 'chikudu kanllu' (literally, 'chicken eyes' - the local term for nightblindness). Bikya took him to a private clinic in Narsampet in May and again in September. On the latter occasion, he spent Rs. 31 for treatment and medicines for Ramesh who had chronic diarrhoea. This was broken down into : Septran syrup (100 mls) Rs. 13; Procain penicillin injection Rs. 5; Vitamin B complex injection Rs. 5; tonic Rs.8. At other times, when the clinics were inacessible, Bikya turned to the local RMP (Registered Medical Practioner) who routinely gave Vitamin B complex injections at Rs. 8 each, and often charged Rs. 10 for tetanus toxoid injections for children with scabies.

Both parents had very low BMI values, with Bikya's being the lowest (15.2) of any man measured. This household was one of 6 in the study population with every household member being malnourished (pattern E). Both Bikya and Jamu often complained of bodily aches and 'weakness'. Jamu was diagnosed by a doctor in a Narsampet clinic early in the year as being severely anaemic and given a course of iron tablets. She claimed her milk dried up 6 months after Ramesh's birth, when she then fed him on cow's milk mixed with rice, and the occasional sorghum 'roti'.

Jamu's aggregate labour participation was higher than the population mean, with the wage labour component particularly high. While she was at work, Ramesh was left in the care of Umballi, who did not appear to be able to cope very well with Ramesh's frequent bouts of diarrhoea, and encouraged him to eat more of the relatively indigestible 'roti' "for strength", than the milk-softened rice. Jamu did not return at midday to feed Ramesh in the rains and at harvest time, when all the family generally omitted a meal. Umballi used to try to feed him some rice left over from breakfast at midday. Ramesh would often be asleep by the time Jamu returned (often at dusk) and finished cooking the evening meal. Jamu and Umballi clearly did not get on well with each other - Jamu appearing to resent her mother-in- laws presence in the home.

In this household, severe malnutrition appears again to have been brought about by a combination of factors but, unlike the first profile household, there was a strong economic facet to this family's problems. The small landholding and the lack of land deeds had caused an extreme dependence on usurious moneylenders and contributed to a situation of household level food shortage. All household members were malnourished, the child severely so.

There were associated non-food factors as well. Ramesh's failure to put on any substantial weight in summer and the rains coincided with regular bouts of illness. Intra-household friction between mother and grandmother, and high levels of maternal labour participation constraining food preparation, also combined to prevent Ramesh growing out of the 'severe' category, despite his weight gains of the latter part of the year.

6.4 SUMMARY

In households containing a severely malnourished child, the compounding effect of the seasonal constraints on maternal time allocation plus the direct effects of relative poverty on food and health expenditure appear to have pushed these households beyond their capacity to cope and precipitated severe malnutrition in one of the more vulnerable members. In a high proportion of households with severe child malnutrition, all the other members show signs of undernutrition - another indicator of household-level food shortage. Severely malnourished children had particularly high rates of disease incidence - an association which was largely independent of household socio-economic status.

It is difficult to say that any one factor is the most crucial in predisposing certain children to severe malnutrition - risk factors interact, each exacerbating the influence of the others. In both of the households profiled, poor growth coincided with seasonally high levels of maternal labour participation and disease incidence among the children. These latter two factors are likely to be inter-related themselves, as the former reduces time available to maintain a healthy environment in the home. In one case there was an additional economic constraint, in the other maternal morbidity may have had an adverse effect on the child. In both cases, the quality of child care given by mother-substitutes to the child was not high.

Note

1. A household with a 4 year old who is not malnourished, may have had a severely malnourished child who died two years previously, or the child him/herself may have been malnourished at an earlier age and experienced sufficient 'catch-up' for the household to be placed in the 'without severe malnutrition' group.

7

CONCLUSIONS

Prior to a discussion of the conclusions of this study, the original central hypothesis is re-iterated:

> *"Within this tribal population, there is insufficient economic inequality for inter-household income differences to be related to child nutritional well-being. Rather, the latter is associated with seasonal peaks in maternal labour participation and child disease incidence."*

In this chapter, each proposition will be dealt with in turn, and the results of the study regarding these will be summarised, prior to a concluding statement on the hypothesis *in toto*. It is outside the scope of this thesis to tackle tribal development and welfare policy thoroughly, but the research does have implications for policy which will be outlined in brief in this chapter.

7.1 What is the Degree of Economic Inequality within this Tribal Community?

Little inequality in the distribution of assets or income was found in the four tribal villages studied here, but socio-economic differences between households were found to exist. Poorer households had larger families, higher economic dependency ratios and smaller landholdings. They were more dependent on labour markets for their income, food markets for their consumption needs and exploitative private moneylenders for credit. A higher proportion of poorer, than richer, households were not eligible for the low-interest institutional bank loans due to their non-possession of land deeds, though there was no discrimination with respect to interest rates in the money market. Income did affect levels of staple calorie consumption of households.

Implications of these results include the need for increased flexibility of bank credit extension to reduce reliance on exploitative non-tribal moneylenders. Low interest loans for all types of farm development, including labour costs could be made available and repayment tied to post-harvest periods, or suspended if the monsoon fails.

The problem of land-deed ownership needs also to be addressed. New land surveys should be carried out and permanent 'pattas' conferred on tribals for the land they cultivate. The Land Transfer Act has to be more strictly enforced to prevent further alienation of tribal land.

7.2 Which Children are Vulnerable to Malnutrition and Ill-health?

With respect to growth retardation amongst under-fives, the three anthropometric indicators differed as to the proportions of children they classified as falling into each category of growth retardation. The weight-for-age indicator classified the most (7.2% and 41.0%), the weight-for-height, the least (0.0% and 10.7%) in the 'severe' and 'moderate' categories respectively. Most children were 'underweight', but stunting was more common than wasting.

Age

A higher proportion of children under 12 months of age, as compared to those between 1 and 5 years, had severe or 'moderate' malnutrition, according to the weight-for-age index. The average age of the eight severely (WA) malnourished children at the beginning of the study period was 9.8 months, with only two children being older than 12 months. Overall and diarrhoeal disease incidence was highest in this age group and the effect of seasonality on nutritional status and disease incidence was particularly marked. The under 12 month age group may have included those children undergoing weaning and those fully breastfed. Both are likely to be particularly at risk when the mother's time is constrained.

Sex

Seven of the eight severely malnourished (WA) children were girls. A much higher proportion of girls than boys in the under 12 month age group were 'moderately' or severely (WA) malnourished, whereas in the other two age groups, proportionately more boys than girls fell into these categories. There appeared to have been a tendency for girls' nutritional status to improve with age, and boys' to deteriorate slightly, according to weight-for-age and height-for- age indices. Girls suffered more from stunting. There were no significant gender differences in the proportions of children with wasting, or acute, malnutrition, according to the weight-for-height index.

Gender differences were not significant either in overall disease incidence, although among girls under 12 months, disease incidence far exceeded that for boys in July - a month of peak female labour demand. This may have contributed to the relatively high prevalence of 'wasting and stunting combined' among girls at this time of the year. In July, the velocity of weight gain among under 12 month old girls was actually negative.

7.3 Are there Seasonal Variations in Child Nutritional and Health Status?

The seasonal dimensions of malnutrition amongst under-fives were quite marked with a peak in the rainy season. Further disaggregation revealed that the most adverse effects on child nutritional status occurred in July, a month during which female labour participation peaked with paddy transplanting. This refines the wet-dry seasonal scenario proposed in Chambers *et al.* (1981) - even data disaggregated by season may mask effects occurring in short recurrent periods of a few weeks. During the rainy season, the lowest seasonal level of household food availability and energy consumption coincided with peaks in child disease incidence and female labour force participation. In contrast, child disease incidence was at its lowest when child nutritional status peaked in winter. These types of seasonal interactions have been reported elsewhere (Schofield 1974; Longhurst and Payne 1979; Chambers 1982; Devkota 1981; Rickleton 1981), though they weren't found to exist in another study in Andhra Pradesh (Ryan *et al.* 1984), probably due to the more widespread use of irrigation there.

There were gender differences in adult perceptions of seasonal vulnerability of the family to ill-health. Women generally regarded the early rains as a critical period, when they were engaged in transplanting, citing child care time constraints as one main reason. Men, on the other hand, saw winter as being an unhealthy time of the year, when they were particularly busy guarding and harvesting crops.

A reduction of marked seasonal fluctuations in nutritional well-being is important, as noted by Chen *et al.* (1979), as these may precipitate more serious forms of deprivation among marginally nourished children than would be the case if smoother seasonal fluctuations could be achieved. Black *et al.* (1984) suggest that because the repeated seasonal checks to growth imposed on a child become progressively less reversible with age, this 'ratcheting' effect is an important mechanism resulting in an accumulation of growth deficits throughout the whole of childhood. Smallness may often come not from some smooth process of steady adaptation, nor in contrast from random shocks, but rather from cyclical periods of relative deprivation and vulnerability (Chambers 1983).

Measures to counteract these seasonal effects might include:

- The government ensuring that each village has at least one functioning borewell before the onset of the rains, when villages are likely to become isolated.
- Locating the health services according to seasonal needs, ensuring adequate staffing and stocking of medicines. The nearest primary health care clinic was too far away for most villagers to risk visiting in the rains, when travel was difficult and the opportunity cost of labour-days foregone greatest.
- Selecting village-level health workers, who do not have to work in the fields, and could also manage creches, possibly incorporating growth monitoring of children, as a means of detecting those children most at risk.
- Government fair-price shops being more accessible and better stocked in the rainy season to reduce seasonal fluctuations in food consumption and reliance on traders selling hoarded paddy at inflated prices.
- The government-run Girijan Corporation, set up to buy minor forest produce from tribals (e.g. tamarind, nuts, honey), at controlled rates, being more accessible to villagers, and accepting small quantities as well as bulk. The tribals' needs for quick returns has often necessitated the sale of small quantities for lower prices at outside markets. This would particularly benefit poorer women who are most involved in this type of work at a time when alternative income- earning opportunities are few.
- One more problematic factor on which action may possibly be considered to ease the seasonal stress for women concerns the timing of pregnancy and child birth, in the light of the conjunction seen between child birth with periods of peak female labour demand, food shortage and high exposure to infection. Discussing desirable times for birth in family welfare programmes may elicit well-founded views women have about

timing of birth, which could lead into questions of how to time and control conceptions.

7.4 Are Inter-household Income Differences Related to Child Nutritional Status?

Despite being positively associated with household calorie consumption, levels of household income did not significantly affect child nutritional status overall in this study area. There were no income-group differences in either the proportions of children suffering different degrees of growth retardation or the seasonality of wasting and stunting. As suggested by Lipton (1983), income is not the sine qua non for the allevation of malnutrition.

However, four of the eight severely weight-for-age malnourished children came from the poorest income group, and none from the richest. Variables reflecting economic poverty were particularly associated with 'severely malnourished households'. Caution should be exercised in attributing a causal link owing to the small cell size involved, although a larger subsample might have revealed a significant inverse relationship between household income and the prevalence of severe child malnutrition.

There were no apparent income differentials in the effect of seasonality on child nutritional status. The children of less affluent households were not more prone to seasonal growth retardation than those from richer households. This again may have been due to the lack of socio-economic inequality in this tribal community, and the fact that there were no differences between household income groups in the levels of aggregate maternal labour participation - a variable shown to have been particularly related to child nutritional status.

Examining proximate food and non-food determinants of malnutrition, no income-group differences in the seasonal variations of child disease incidence were found, but seasonality did have a greater impact on aggregate calorie consumption in poorer households. Poorer households were more likely to have had dwindling food stocks in the rains, when fair price shops were relatively inaccessible, and transport of purchases difficult. Several households particularly poorer ones, more dependent on wage labour, cut out one meal per day in the rainy season, while winter was the season of relative plenty after the paddy harvest.

7.5 Are Child Nutritional Status and Morbidity Inter-related?

The particularly strong association between child morbidity and severe child malnutrition was independent of the socio-economic status of the household; a finding similar to other studies (Watson 1984; Victora *et al.* 1986). As noted by several researchers (Taylor *et al.* 1978; Abdullah 1983; Lipton 1983; Hassan and Ahmad 1984; Payne 1985), the impact of disease may be such as not only to overlay but to extensively distort the effects that variations in food availability would otherwise have. Improvements in the quality of the environment e.g. water supplies, housing, general sanitation may be more likely to have a positive impact on child nutritional status, through improving child health, than raising the food intake of children living in poor environmental conditions, as contended by some medical doctors and nutritionists (Margen 1981; Ryan *et al.* 1984).

7.6 Is Child Nutritional Status associated with Maternal Labour Participation and Time Allocation?

Similar to some findings (Kumar 1978; Popkin 1980), but contrary to more (Blau 1981; Tripp 1981; Smith *et al.* 1983; Ryan *et al.* 1984), maternal labour participation was found to be inversely related to child nutritional status, despite the increased levels of income earned by the mother. The need for a particularly high female work input in the paddy transplanting month of July, at a time of peak disease incidence in children, and low household food availability, resulted in the most severe mean infant growth retardation occurring in this month. A consequence of female labour demand peaking at this time is a reduction in the efficacy of child care and feeding. High female labour force participation was virtually universal, though women from the richest income group did tend to work fewer days per month on average; except, that is, in the early rainy season months of June and July.

Strategies aimed at the amelioration of womens' work loads at particular times should be pursued. As pointed out by the ILO (1976), in rural areas, "most women in developing countries are overworked rather than underemployed, and a more appropriate technology for the tasks they perform implies labour saving.....rather than employment creation". Various possibilities have been suggested to lighten the disproportionate work burdens that fall on women, especially during times of peak labour demand (Palmer 1981).

Examples are appropriate technologies for transplanting and post-harvest processing, improved water supplies (which relieve women of longer journeys carrying water) and improved hoes which reduce the energy used in weeding. Care is required to ensure that this does not take the form of displacement of labour from paid work. The emphasis, rather, needs to be on reducing drudgery in unpaid tasks, e.g. food processing, cooking, cleaning, fetching water and gathering fuel.

Other possibilities include the revision of work organisation to allow for breastfeeding and child care or the establishment of child care facilities in seasons of stress. As womens' seasonal work in this area is characterised by gang labour, the potential for collective child care is obvious. Day care or creche facilities may also be a suitable location for seasonal child feeding, particularly as household food availability is low at a time when child care is most needed. This has been done successfully in several places e.g. harvest season day-care centres were an effective addition to the Narangwal Project child health programme in the Punjab, North India (Chambers 1982).

The government agency responsible for initiating and implementing tribal development schemes, the Integrated Tribal Development Agency (ITDA), annually delivers sacks of child feeding mixture to these tribal villages. These would be most useful if timed to arrive in June or July (rather than the summer months when they are normally sent), when time available to the mother for food preparation is particularly constrained.

These interventions, however, are all extra-household and do not take into account intra-household power relations behind gender- typing the total household work load, or how altering this might also contribute to ameliorating womens' work burdens. Patriarchy is likely to be the main obstacle to securing a fairer distribution of work between adult household members. This effect is likely to be most pronounced in this study area in the richest households where there was more gender bias in decision-making power. For example, there might have been resistance by richer household heads to a strategy of using hired labour to alleviate high on-farm work loads.

Palmer (1981) has suggested possible ways for women to negotiate an easier work load and demand appropriate technologies e.g. the reform of rural institutions (especially farming co-operatives) to allow women full membership rights and direct access to the returns to their household labour. The function of a farmer's co-operative could also be extended to imposing a levy on household income from the sale of produce to finance investment in some technology which reduces womens' work load in unremunerated tasks.

7.7 SUMMARY

In terms of the central hypothesis, there appears to have been sufficient economic inequality to affect the calorie consumption of poorer households vis-a-vis richer ones. There were, however, no significant income differentials overall for the study community, in the prevalence, severity or seasonality of child growth retardation. Total household income per CU was not linearly associated with child nutritional status.

Aggregate maternal labour participation, however, had a significant inverse relationship with the nutritional status of young children, which was independent of the level of household income.

Seasonality was important through its effect of intensifying the conflict between the maternal need to maintain household food security (through agricultural work) on the one hand, and the competing demands for child care on the other. This dilemma was particularly serious in the early rainy season when both female labour demand and child morbidity peaked. At this time of the year, child nutritional status was generally at its lowest level. Thus, considering the nutritional well-being of children from the whole study community, the hypothesis appears to have been upheld. There are, however, some important qualifications.

Aggregating the results for children with varying degrees of growth retardation appears to have masked the existence of poverty-related characteristics in most of the households with severely malnourished children. The absence of severe child malnutrition in the richest income group and its existence in nearly 1 in 4 households from the poorest group indicates how richer households appear to have the means - in the form of available food or income for food or health - to buffer themselves from the more serious effects of the maternal conflict between household food security and child care, unlike some of the poorer households. Furthermore, a high proportion of 'severely malnourished households' exhibited intra- household anthropometric patterns indicative of household-level food shortage.

REFERENCES

Abdullah, M. (1983) Dimensions of Intra Household Food and Nutrient Allocation: A Study of a Bangladeshi Village. PhD. thesis, University of London.

Aguillon, D.B., Caedo, N.M., Arnold, J.C. and Engel, R.W. (1982) The Relationship of Family Characteristics to the Nutritional Status of Pre-School Children. Food and Nutrition Bulletin, 4 (4), 5-12.

Athreya, V.B. (1985) 'Gangaikondan 1916-1984: Change and Stability'. Working Paper No. 56, Madras Institute of Development Studies, Madras.

Bailey, K.V. (1965) Quality and Composition of Breastmilk in some New Guinean Populations. Journal of Tropical Pediatrics, 11, 35.

Bairagi, R. (1980) Is Income the only Constraint on Child Nutrition in Rural Bangladesh ?. Bulletin of the World Health Organisation, 58 (5), 767-772.

Bairagi, R. (1983) Dynamics of Child Nutrition in Rural Bangladesh. Ecology of Food and Nutrition, 13, 173-178.

Bairagi, R., Chowdhury, M.K., Young, J.K. and Curlin, G.T. (1985) Alternative Anthropometric Indicators of Mortality. American Journal of Clinical Nutrition, 42, 296-306.

Bandopadhyay, A. (1979) The Status of Landholders in Tribal Bihar. Mimeo.

Bardhan, K. (1987) Women's Work, Welfare and Status. Economic and Political Weekly, 20 (50), 2207-2220 ; 20 (51-2), 2261-69.

Baumgartner, R.N. and Pollit, E. (1983) The Bacon Chow Study: Analysis of the Effects of Infectious Illnesses on the Growth of Infants. Nutrition Research, 3 9-21.

Becker, S., Black, R.E., Brown, K.H. and Nahar, S. (1986) Relations between Socio-Economic Status and Morbidity, Food Intake and Growth in Young Children in Two Villages in Bangladesh. Ecology of Food and Nutrition, 18, 251-264.

Beteille, A. (1974) Six Essays in Comparative Sociology Oxford University Press, New Delhi.

Bhan, M.K., Arora, N.K., Ghai, O P., Ramachandran, K., Khoshoo, V. and Bhandari, N. (1986) Major Factors in Diarrhoea Related Mortality among Rural Children. Indian Journal of Medical Research, 83, 9-12.

Bharadwaj, K. (1974) Production Conditions in Indian Agriculture. Cambridge University Press.

Bhuiya, A., Wojtyniak, B., D'Souza, S. and Zimicki, S. (1986) Socio-economic Determinants of Child Nutritional Status: Boys versus Girls. Food and Nutrition Bulletin, 8 (3), 3-7.

Bidinger, P.D., Nag, B. and Babu, P. (1986) Nutritional and Health Consequences of Seasonal Fluctuations in Household Food Availability. Food and Nutrition Bulletin, 8 (1), 36-60.

Black, R.E., Brown, K.H. and Becker, S. (1984) Malnutrition is a Determining Factor in Diarrhoeal Duration, but not in Incidence, Among Rural Children in a Longitudinal Study in Rural Bangladesh. American Journal of Clinical Nutrition, Vol. 37, 87-94.

Blau, D.M. (1981) Investments in Child Nutrition and Women's Allocation of Time in Developing Countries. Discussion Paper 371. New Haven, Conn., USA: Yale University, Economic Growth Center.

Briend, A., Dykewicz, C., Graven, K., Mazumder, R.N., Wojtyniak, B. and Bennish, M. (1986) Usefulness of Nutritional Indices and Classifications in Predicting Death of Malnourished Children. British Medical Journal, 293, 373-75.

Briscoe, J. (1979) The Quantitative Effect of Infection on the Use of Food by Young Infants in Poor Countries. American Journal of Clinical Nutrition, 32, 648-676.

Brown, K.H., Black, R.E. and Becker, S. (1982) Seasonal Changes in Nutritional Status and the Prevalence of Malnutrition in a Longitudinal Study of Young Children in Rural Bangladesh. American Journal of Clinical Nutrition, 36, 303.

Bryceson, D. (1980) Proletarianisation of Tanzanian Women. Review of African Political Economy, No. 17.

Byres, T. (1981) The New Technology, Class Formation and Class Action in the Indian Countryside. Journal of Peasant Studies, 8 (4).

Caldwell, P. and Caldwell, J. (1987) Where there is a Narrower Gap between Female and Male Situations: Lessons from South India and Sri Lanka. Dhaka, BAMENEH / American SSRC Workshop on Excess Female Mortality, mimeo.

Carloni, A.S. (1981) Sex Disparities in Distribution of Food within Rural Households. Food and Nutrition, 7, 3-12.

Chambers, R., Longhurst, R. and Pacey, A. (eds). (1981) Seasonal Dimensions to Rural Poverty, Francis Pinter, London.

Chambers, R. (1982) Health, Agriculture and Rural Poverty: Why Seasons Matter. Journal of Development Studies, 18 (2), 217-238.

Chambers, R. (1983) Seasonality, Poverty and Nutrition: A Professional Frontier. Paper presented at the EFNAG National Workshop on Poverty and Malnutrition, 7-10 February, Tamil Nadu Agricultural University, Coimbatore, India.

Chambers, R. (1987) Poverty in India: Concepts, Research and Reality, mimeo.

Chayanov, A.V. (1966) The Theory of Peasant Economy. Homewood, Ill. Richard D. Irwin.

Chen, L.C., Ahmed, S., Gesche, M. and Mosley, W.H. (1974) A Prospective Study of Birth Interval Dynamics in Rural Bangladesh. Population Studies, 28, 277.

Chen, L.C., Chowdhury, A.K.M.A. and Huffman, S.L. (1979) Seasonal Dimensions of Energy Protein Malnutrition in Rural Bangladesh: the Role of Agriculture, Dietary Practices and Infection. Ecology of Food and Nutrition, 8, 175.

Chen, L.C., Chowdhury, A.K.M.A. and Huffman, S.L. (1980) Anthropometric Assessment of Energy Protein Malnutrition and the Subsequent Risk of Mortality among Pre-School Aged Children. American Journal of Clinical Nutrition, 33, 1836-1845.

Chen, L.C., Huq, e. and D'Souza, S. (1981) Sex Bias in the Allocation of Food and Family Health Care in Rural Bangladesh. Population and Development Review, 7 (1), 55-70.

Chimwaza, B.N. (1982) Food and Nutrition in Malawi. PhD. thesis, University of London.

Clark, A.W. (1987) The Social Demography of Excess Female Mortality in India: New Directions. Paper prepared for the BAMENEH / American SSRC Workshop on Excess Female Mortality, Dhaka, January 1987.

Corbridge, S. (1986) State, Tribe and Region: Policy and Politics in India's Jharkhand, 1900-1980. Phd. thesis, University of Cambridge.

Corbridge, S. (1988) The Ideology of Tribal Economy and Society: Politics in the Jharkhand, 1950-1980. Modern Asian Studies, 22 (1), 1-42.

Crookes, N. and Dyson, T. (1981) Data on Seasonality of Births and Deaths. In: Chambers, R. *et al.* (eds) Seasonal Dimensions to Rural Poverty, Francis Pinter, London.

Da Corta (1988) Famines and Peasant Mobility in South India, DPhil. thesis, Oxford University.

Dandekar V.M. and Rath N. (1971) Poverty in India. Indian School of Political Economy, Delhi.

Das Gupta, M. (1987) The Second Daughter: Sex Differentials in Child Mortality, Nutrition and Health Care in Punjab, North India. Paper prepared for the BAMANEH/American SSRC Workshop on Excess Female Mortality, Dhaka, 1987.

De Chavez, M.M., Arroyo, P., Gil, S.E.P., Hernandez, M., Quiroz, S.E., Rodriguez, M., De Hermelo, M.P. and Chavez, A. (1974) The Epidemiology of Good Nutrition in a Population with a high Prevalence of Malnutrition'. Ecology of Food Nutrition, 3, 223-230.

Deere, C.D. and de Janvry, A. (1979) A Conceptual Framework for the Empirical Analysis of Peasants. American Journal of Agricultural Economics, November, 601-11.

Devkota, S. (1981) Monitoring Rural Development with Nutritional Status Assessment. MSc. thesis, Department of Human Nutrition, London School of Hygiene and Tropical Medicine.

Dubos, R. (1985) Mirage of Health. In: Black, N. *et al.* (eds) Health and Disease: a Reader, Open University Press.

Dugdale, A.E. (1985) Family Anthropometry: A New Strategy for Determining Community Nutrition. The Lancet, 21 September, 672.

Dugdale, A.E. (1987), A Weight for Height Index for Adolescents'. LSHTM mimeo.

Edholm, F., Harris, O. and Young, K. (1977) Conceptualising Women. Critique of Anthropology, Vol. 3, No. 9/10.

FAO/WHO/UNU. (1985) Energy and Protein Requirements. Report of a Joint FAO/WHO/UNU Expert Consultation. WHO Technical Report Series, No.724, Geneva.

FAO/WHO. (1973) Energy and Protein Requirements. Report of a joint FAO/WHO ad hoc expert committee, March 22-April 2, 1971. FAO

Nutrition Meetings Report Series No. 522, Rome, Italy; Geneva, Switzerland WHO.

Ferro-Luzzi, A., James, W.P.T. and Waterlow, J.C. (1988) The Definition of Chronic Energy Deficiency. Mimeo.

Gillespie, S.R. (1983) Commodity Exchange Relations and the Effect of Seasonality in the Kovilpatti Region of South India. MSc. thesis, Department of Human Nutrition, London School of Hygiene and Tropical Medicine.

Gomez, F., Galvan, R., Cravioto, J., and Frenck, S. (1955) Malnutrition in Infancy and Childhood, with special reference to kwashiorkor. Advances in Paediatrics, 7, 131-136.

Gopalan, C. and Narasingarao B.S. (1971) Dietary Allowances for Indians. ICMR Special Report No. 66. Delhi.

Gopaldas, T. (1983) The Impact of Programmes, Projects and Policies on Malnutrition in India. In: Kennedy, E.T. and Pinstrup-Andersen, P. Nutrition Related Policies and Programmes, IFPRI, Washington.

Grantham-McGregor, S. (1984) The Social Background of Childhood Malnutrition. In Malnutrition and Behaviour: Critical Assessment of Key Issues, Nestle Foundation Publication Series, Vol. 4, 358-374.

Grewal, T. Gopaldas, T. and Gadre, V.J. (1973) Etiology of Malnutrition in Rural Indian Pre-School Children (Madhya Pradesh). Environmental Child Health, 265-270.

Gupta, S. and Srivastava, G. (1977) Childhood Morbidity in relation to number of Children in Unitary and Joint Families. Indian Paediatrics, 14, 837-840.

Guyer, J.I. (1986) Intra-Household Processes and Farming Systems Research: Perspectives from Anthropology. In: Joyce Lewinger Moock (ed.) Understanding Africa's Rural Households and Farming Systems, Boulder and London: Westview Press, 92-104.

Haaga, J.G. and Mason, J.B. (1987) Food Distribution within the Family: Evidence and Implications for Research and Programmes. Food Policy, May, 146-160.

Hanumantha Rao, D. and Satyanarayana, K. (1974) Nutritional Status of Tribal Pre-School Children of Andhra Pradesh. Indian Journal of Nutrition and Dietetics, 11, 328.

Harriss, B. (1983) Exchange Relations and Poverty in Dryland Agriculture. Concept Publishing Co., Delhi.

Harriss, B. (1987a) Poverty in India: Micro-Level Evidence. Paper presented at the Workshop on Poverty in India, Queen Elizabeth House, Oxford, October 1987.

Harriss, B. (1987b) Differential Female Mortality and Health Care in South Asia. Report of a Conference held in Dacca, Bangladesh in January 1987 and organised jointly by the South Asian Committee of the American Social Science Research Council and the Bangladesh Association for Maternal and Neonatal Health.

Hassan, N. and Ahmad, K. (1984) Intra-Familial Distribution of food in Rural Bangladesh. Food and Nutrition Bulletin, 6 (4), 34-42.

Henry, F. (1981) Environmental Sanitation and Nutritional Status Infants in Rural St. Lucia, West Indies. Trans. Roy. Soc. Trop. Med. Hyg., 75 (4), 507.

Hernandez, M., Perez Hidalgo, C., Ramirez Hernandez, J., Madrigal, H. and Chavez, A. (1974) Effect of Economic Growth on Nutrition in a Tropical Community. Ecology of Food and Nutrition, 3, 283-291.

Heywood, P.F. (1986) Nutritional Status as a Risk Factor for Mortality in Children in the Highlands of Papua New Guinea. In: Proceedings of the XIII International Congress of Nutrition, Taylor, T.G. and Jenkins, N.K. (eds) pp. 103-106; John Libbey, London

Hilder, A.S. and Steinhoff, M.C. (1983) RUHSA Nutritional Status and Immunisation Survey: Preliminary Report. CMC Hospital, Vellore, South

India.

Hill, P. (1982) Dry Grain Farming Families. Cambridge University Press, London.

Howard, G.R. (1978) Socio-economic Factors affecting Utilization of a Rural Indian Hospital. Tropical Doctor, 211-19.

International Labour Office. (1976) Employment, Growth and Basic Needs: a One-World Problem, Geneva, ILO.

Jeffery, P., Jeffery, R. and Lyon, A. (1987) Domestic Politics and Sex Differences in Mortality: a view from rural Bijnor District, U.P. Paper prepared for the BAMENEH / American SSRC Workshop on Excess Female Mortality, Dhaka, mimeo.

Jelliffe, D.B. (1966) The Assessment of the Nutritional Status of the Community. Monograph Series 53, Geneva, WHO.

Jodha, N.S. (1983) Market Forces and the Erosion of Common Property Resources. Paper presented at the International Workshop on Agricultural Markets in the Semi-Arid Tropics, ICRISAT Center, Andhra Pradesh, India 24-28 October 1983.

Kasongo Project Team (1986) Growth Decelerations among Under Five Year Old Children in Kasongo (Zaire). II Relationship with Subsequent Risk of Dying, and Operational Consequences. Bulletin of the WHO, 64, 703-09.

Keilmann, A.A. and McCord, C. (1978) Weight-for-age as an Index of Risk of Death in Children. Lancet, 1, 1247-1250.

Kirkwood, B. R. (1988) Essentials of Medical Statistics, Blackwell Scientific Publications: Oxford.

Koenig, M. and D'Souza (1986) Sex Differences in Child Mortality in rural Bangladesh. Social Science and Medicine, 22 (1), 15-22.

Keller, W. (1983) Choice of Indicators of Nutritional Status. In

Evaluation of Nutrition Education in Third World Communities, Hans Huber Publishers, Vienna.

Kumar, S.K. (1978) Role of Household Economy in Child Nutrition at Low Incomes: A Case Study in Kerala. Occasional Paper No. 95, Dept. of Agricultural Economics, Cornell University.

Kumar, S.K. (1983) A Framework for Tracing Policy Effects on Intra-household Food Distribution. Food and Nutrition Bulletin, Vol. 5, No. 4, 13-16.

Kutumbaiah, P. (1969) Ancient Indian Medicine, Orient Longmans, Bombay.

Kynch, J. and McGuire, M. (1986) Report on the Nutritional Status of Families in Palanpur, U.P., India. Oxford mimeo.

Levinson, J.F. (1978) "Morinda": An Economic Analysis of Malnutrition Among Young Children in Rural India., Cornell/MIT International Policy Series, Cambridge, USA.

Lipton, M. (1983) Poverty, Undernutrition and Hunger, World Bank Staff Working Paper No. 597, Washington D.C.

Longhurst, R. and Payne, P.R. (1979) Seasonal Aspects of Nutrition: A Review of Evidence and Policy Implications. IDS Discussion Paper, 145., Institute of Development Studies, Sussex, U.K.

Mackintosh, M. (1981) Gender and Economics: The Sexual Division of Labour and the Subordination of Women. In: Of Marriage and the Market, edited by Young, K., Wolkowitz, C. and McCullagh, R. CSE Books.

Margen, S. (1981): Retrospective Reactions. Report of the Summer Institute on Newer Concepts in Nutrition and Health and their Implications for Social Policy, 16 March - 4 April, 1981. Pune, India. Maharasthra Association for Cultivation of Science.

Martorell, R., Yarbrough, C., Yarbrough, S. and Klein, R.E. (1980) The Impact of Ordinary Illnesses on the Dietary Intakes of Malnourished

Children. American Journal of Clinical Nutrition, 33, 345-350.

Martorell, R. Leslie, J. and Moock, P.R. (1984) Characteristics and Determinants of Child Nutritional Status in Nepal. American Journal of Clinical Nutrition 39, 74-86.

Mata, L.J. Kromal, R.A., Urrutia, J.J. and Garcia, B. (1977) Effect of Infection on Food Intake and the Nutritional State: Perspectives as Viewed from a Village. American Journal of Clinical Nutrition, 30, 1215-1227.

McNeill G. (1985) Energy Undernutrition in Adults in Rural South India; RUHSA/LSHTM Nutrition Research Project Progress Report, London School of Hygiene and Tropical Medicine, mimeo.

Mudkhedkar, S.N. and Shah, P.M. (1976) The Effect of Spacing of Children on the Nutrition and Mortality of Under-Fives. Indian Journal of Medical Research, 64 (7), 953-958.

Mukherjee, D.K. and Sethna, N.J. (1972) The Ecology of Growth in Under-Privileged Children. Indian Paediatrics, 9, 440-446.

Murrillo, S. (1983) The Effects of Social Factors on the Nutritional Status of Urban Costa Rican Children. PhD. Thesis, University of London.

Nabarro D. (1984) Social, Economic, Health and Environmental Determinants of Nutritional Status: A Case Study from Nepal, Food and Nutrition Bulletin, 6, 1, 18-32.

Nadkarni, M.V. (1980) Marketable Surplus and Market Dependence in a Millet Region, Allied, Delhi.

National Institute of Nutrition, Hyderabad, India. Weight and Height Standards for Boys and Girls. In: Ryan, J.G., *et al.*, The Determinants of Individual Diets and Nutritional Status in Six Villages of Southern India. ICRISAT Research Bulletin No. 7, 1984.

NIN (1984) Nutritive Value of Indian Foods, National Institute of

Nutrition: Hyderabad.

NIN (1986) Annual Report 1985-86, National Institute of Nutrition Hyderabad.

National Nutrition Monitoring Bureau (1981) Report for the year 1980, National Institute of Nutrition: Hyderabad.

NCHS Growth Curves for Children, Birth-18 years, United States. Rockville M.D. National Center for Health Statistics, 1977. Vital and Health Statistics, Series 11, No. 165; DHEW.

Pacey, A. and Payne, P. (eds) (1985) Agricultural Development and Nutrition. Hutchinson.

Palmer, I. (1981) Seasonal Dimensions of Women's Roles. In: Chambers, R. *et al.* (eds) Seasonal Dimensions to Rural Poverty, Francis Pinter, London.

Patnaik, U. (1976) Class Differentiation within the Peasantry: An Approach to Analysis of Indian Agriculture. Economic and Political Weekly, Sep., A82-A102.

Payne, P.R. (1985) Public Health and Functional Consequences of Seasonal Hunger and Malnutrition. Paper prepared for Workshop on Seasonal Causes of Food Insecurity, Policy Implications and Research Needs, London School of Hygiene and Tropical Medicine, mimeo.

Perera, D.A. (1983) The Nutritional Status Surveys of Preschool Children in Sri Lanka. 14-51. In Government of Sri Lanka (1983) Nutritional Status: its Determinants and Intervention Programmes. Colombo Food and Nutrition Policy and Planning Division, Ministry of Plan Implementation.

Plattner, S. (1974) Wealth and Growth among Mayan Peasants. Human Ecology, Vol. 2, 75-87.

Poleman, T.T. (1981) Quantifying the Nutrition Situation in Developing Countries. Food Research Institute Studies, 18 (1), 1-58.

Popkin, B.M. and Solon, F.S. (1976) Income, Time, the Working Mother and Child Nutriture. Environmental Child Health, August 1976, 156.

Popkin, B.M. (1980) Time Allocation of the Mother and Child Nutrition. Ecology of Food and Nutrition, 9, 1-14.

Prahlad Rao, N. (1980) Determinants of Nutritional Status in India. In: Binswanger, H.P. *et al.* (eds) Rural Household Studies in Asia. Singapore University Press.

Prasad, P.H., Rodgers, G.B., Gupta, S., Sharma, A.N. and Sharma, B. (1986) The Pattern of Poverty in Bihar. Population and Labour Policies Programme Working Paper, No. 152, World Employment Programme, ILO, Geneva.

Rahman, A. (1986) Peasants and Classes: a Study in Differentiation in Bangladesh. Zed Books: London.

Raikes, P. (1981) Seasonality in Rural Economy. In: Chambers, R. *et al.* (eds) Seasonal Dimensions to Rural Poverty, Francis Pinter, London.

Rajagopalan, S. and Kymal, P.K. (1981) Births, Work and Nutrition in Tamil Nadu, India. In: Chambers, R. *et al.* (eds) Seasonal Dimensions to Rural Poverty, Francis Pinter, London.

Ramachandran, V.K. (1986) Socio-economic character of Agrarian Labour in a Vanguard Agrarian Region: a Case Study of Gokilapuram Village, Madurai District. PhD. thesis, Madras.

Ramaiah, P. (1981) Tribal Economy of India, Light and Life Publishers, New Delhi.

Rawson, I. and Valverde, V. (1976) The Aetiology of Malnutrition among Pre-School Children in Rural Costa Rica. Journal of Tropical Pediatrics and Environmental Child Health, 22, 12.

Rickleton, J. (1981) Nutrition and Agriculture in East Nepal. MSc. thesis, Department of Human Nutrition, London School of Hygiene and Tropical Medicine.

Rowland, M.G.M. Cole, T.J. and Whitehead, R.G. (1977) A Quantitative Study into the Role of Infection in Determining Nutritional Status in Gambian Village Children. British Journal of Nutrition, 37, 441-450.

Ryan, J.G. Bidinger, P.D., Prahlad Rao, N. and Pushpamma, P. (1984) The Determinants of Individual Diets and Nutritional Status in Six Villages of South India., Research Bulletin No. 7. ICRISAT Economics Programme, Hyderabad.

Schofield, S. (1974) Seasonal Factors affecting Nutrition In Different Age Groups and especially Pre-School Children. Journal of Development Studies, 11 (1), 22-40.

Scrimshaw, N.S. Taylor, C.E. and Gordon, J.E. (1968) Interactions of Nutrition and Infection, WHO Monograph Series No. 37.

Seckler, D. (1981) Optimal Body Size and a Possible Production Constant. Ford Foundation, New Delhi, mimeo.

Sen, A. (1981) Poverty and Famines: An Essay on Entitlement and Deprivation, Clarendon Press, Oxford.

Sen, A. (1984) Resources, Values and Development, Blackwell, Oxford.

Shaikh, K. and Becker, S. (1985) Socioeconomic Status and Fertility in Rural Bangladesh. Journal of Biosocial Sciences, 17, 81-89.

Shatrugna, M. (1985) Myth of Minimum Wages for Agricultural Labour. Economic and Political Weekly, May, 871-72.

Shears, E. (1982) Aspects of Seasonality in Two Dryland Agricultural Villages of India. MSc. thesis, Dept. of Human Nutrition, London School of Hygiene and Tropical Medicine.

Smith, M.F. Paulsen, S.K., Fougere, W. and Ritchey, S.J. (1983) Socio-economic Education and Health Factors influencing Growth of Rural Haitian Children. Ecology of Food and Nutrition, 13, 99-108.

SPSS Inc. (1983) SPSSx Users Guide, McGraw-Hill Book Company,

Massachusetts.

Stini, W. (1981) Body Composition and Nutrient Reserves in Evolutionary Perspective. World Review of Nutrition and Dietetics, 37, 55-83.

Stinson, S. (1983) Socioeconomic Status and Child Growth in Rural Bolivia. Ecology of Food and Nutrition, 13, 179-187.

Sukhatme, P.V. (1981) Relationship between Malnutrition and Poverty. Mimeo, First National Conference on Social Sciences, National Council of Applied Economic Research, New Delhi.

Taylor, C.A. Emanuel, I., Morris, L.N. and Prosterman, R.L. (1978) Child Nutrition in the Phillipines: Is Socio-Economic Status Important ?. Tropical Pediatrics and Environmental Child Health, April, 80-86.

Thompson, B. and Rahaman, A.K. (1967) Infant Feeding and Child Care in a West African Village. Journal of Tropical Pediatrics, 13, 124.

Timmer, C.P. Falcon, W.P. and Pearson, S.R. (1983) Food Policy Analysis. The John Hopkins University Press for the World Bank, Baltimore and London.

Tomkins, A.M., Drasar, B.S., Bradley, A.K. and Williamson, W.A. (1978): Water Supply and Nutritional Status in Rural Northern Nigeria. Trans. Roy. Soc. Trop. Med. Hyg., Vol. 72, No. 3, 239.

Tomkins, A.M. (1983) Nutritional Cost of Protracted Diarrhoea in Young Gambian Children. GUT, 24, 459.

Tomkins, A.M. (1986) Protein Energy Malnutrition and the Risk of Infection. Proceedings of the Nutrition Society, Vol. 45, No. 3, 289- 304.

Tomkins, A. and Watson, F. (1988) Interaction of Nutrition and Infection: a Review. LSHTM mimeo.

Tripp, R.B. (1981) Farmers and Traders: Some Economic Determinants of Nutritonal Status In Northern Ghana. Journal of Tropical Pediatrics,

27, 15-22.

UNICEF. (1981) Socio-economic Characteristics of Functional Groups of Malnourished Populations in Costa Rica. Social Statistics Bulletin, East African Regional Office (UNICEF), Vol 4, No. 4, 9.

Valverde, V. Martorell, R., Mejia-Pivaral, V., Delgado, H., Lechtig, A., Teller, C. and Klein, R.E. (1977) The Relationship between Family Land Availability and Nutritional Status. Ecology of Food and Nutrition, 6, 1-7.

Victora, C.G., Vaughan, J.P., Kirkwood, B.R., Martines, J.C. and Barcelos, L.B. (1986) Risk Factors for Malnutrition in Brazilian Children: the Role of Social and Environmental Variables. Bulletin of WHO, Vol. 64, No. 2, 299-309.

Von Furer-Haimendorf, C. (1982) Tribes of India: The Struggle for Survival. University of California Press, Ltd., London.

Walsh, R.P.D. (1981) The Nature of Climatic Seasonality. In: Chambers, R., *et al.* (eds) Seasonal Dimensions to Rural Poverty, Francis Pinter London.

Warrier, S. (1987) Daughter Disfavour, Women, Work and Autonomy in Rural West Bengal. Paper prepared for the BAMENEH / American SSRC Workshop on Excess Female Mortality, Dhaka.

Waterlow, J.C. (1972) Classification and Definition of Protein- Calorie Malnutrition. British Medical Journal, No. 3, 566-69.

Waterlow, J.C. Buzina, R., Keller, W., Lane, J.M., Nichaman, M.Z. and Tanner, J.M. (1977) The Presentation and Use of Height and Weight Data for Comparing the Nutritional Status of Groups of Children under the Age of 10 Years. Bulletin of WHO, 55, 489-498.

Watson, E. (1984) The Relationship between Undernutrition and Indebtedness in Four Villages in Tissamaharama, Sri Lanka. London School of Hygiene and Tropical Medicine, mimeo.

Watson, E. and Harriss, B. (1985) Health, Nutrition and Work: A Review of Relationships of Discrimination against Women in South Asia. Discussion Paper No. 179, School of Development Studies, University of East Anglia.

White, B. (1980) Rural Household Studies in Anthropological Persective. In: Binswanger *et al.* (eds) Rural Household Studies in Asia, Singapore University Press, 3-25.

White, B. (1984) Measuring Time Allocation, Decision-Making and Agrarian Changes affecting Rural Women: Examples from Recent Research in Indonesia. IDS Bulletin, 15 (1), 18-32.

Whitehead, A. (1981) I'm Hungry, Mum: The Politics of Domestic Budgetting In: Young, K. *et al.* (eds), 1981. Of Marriage and the Market: Women's Subordination in International Perspective, CSE Books, London.

WHO. (1983) Measuring Change in Nutritional Status, World Health Organisation, Geneva.

Wolfe, B.L. and Behrman, J.R. (1982) Determinants of Child Mortality, Health and Nutrition in a Developing Country. Journal of Development Economics, 11, 163-193.

Wray, J.D. and Aguirre, A. (1969) Protein Calorie Malnutrition in Candelaria, Columbia. I. Prevalence, Social and Demographic Causal Factors, Journal of Tropical Pediatrics, September, 76-98.

Zeitlin, M. (1985) Positive Deviance in Young Children in Developing Countries ; Report to UNICEF (draft).

APPENDIX I

CLASSIFICATION OF HOUSEHOLDS BY ENTITLEMENT

To investigate the efficacy of the entitlement concept as a means of classification, households were classified according to the available sources of income comprising their entitlement bases. The table below describes the five groups that emerged.

TABLE A1 : Household entitlement bases

Entitlement group income sources	No. households	Total household income per CU (Rs.)	% income from exchange
Wage labour	3	894	100.0
Wage labour Crop production	45	1502	54.2
Wage labour Crop production Others (non-agric.)	1	1581	44.9
Wage labour Crop production Livestock	13	1719	49.8
Wage labour Crop production Livestock Others (non-agric.)	5	2127	61.4

The poorest households in group 1, were landless and dependent entirely on wage labour. There was a significant negative association between total household income per CU and the percentage of income derived from exchange (r=-0.34; P<0.01), indicating an increasing dependence on the exchange entitlement as household income decreases. The richest households were those whose sources of income were most diverse, though only 5 households fell into this category (group 5), and the mean income was largely contributed to by the relatively large temporary salaries paid to two individuals, by bidi-leaf contractors, to act as middlemen. In terms of total household income per CU, one-way analysis of variance techniques revealed no significant differences between entitlement groups (P=0.73). The percentage income derived from exchange entitlement (where exchange refers to the sale of crops, livestock products and labour), varied from 100% (landless) to 45% , though in landed households the range of variation was not large (16.5%).

The entitlement concept has been used here in a descriptive fashion, as a means of characterising the population, in this case with respect to the structure of production and exchange. It has, however, shown a degree of homogeneity between households with respect to the type of income source available.

It is interesting to note the near significance (P=0.07) of income-group differences in the percentage income from exchange, as revealed by oneway analysis of variance. Thus, the income classification used actually does differentiate households empirically quite well on the basis of their E-mapping.

APPENDIX II

METHOD FOR CALCULATING CONSUMPTION UNITS

The technique of converting household to consumption units (CUs), based on caloric recommendations, is simple and allows one to standardise households of varying size, age and sex distribution for cross-comparison purposes. Consumption units should be used in a relative sense. Individual requirements of family members cannot be aggregated without making assumptions about distribution in addition to those which have been made in order to fix the requirements of each of the members (Payne 1985).

Many nutrition studies carried out in the past in India have used the Indian Council of Medical Research (ICMR) allowances as the basis for consumption unit coefficient calculations (Gopalan and Narasingarao 1971). These are based on the energy requirement of a moderately active man weighing 55 kg., and are as follows :

Age (years)	Sex	kcal./day	CU
>15 (adult)	M	2800	1.00
>15 (adult)	F	2300	0.82
10-14	M	2300	0.82
10-14	F	2100	0.75
6-9	M+F	1800	0.64
<5	M+F	1350	0.48

The energy requirements of adult men and women in the study community were estimated using the FAO/WHO/UNU method (1985). This entailed calculating the basal metabolic rate (BMR) of a man and woman of average weight and height, using predictive equations. Next, the BMR value was multiplied by a coefficient relating to the average level of daily activity of a man and woman. Time allocation data was used to determine the average time spent in various types of activity, with various energy costs. The mean energy cost (as a multiple of BMR) of daily activity for men and women was then calculated as an average of the energy costs of all daily activities, weighted with respect to the number of hours actually spent in each type of activity.

For example, the BMR of a woman of average weight (43.2 kg.) and average height (1.52 m.) was calculated as being 1117 kcals. and the daily activity index was calculated as being 2.0, giving a daily energy requirement of 2234 kcals. Likewise, for men of average weight (49.9 kg.) and height (1.66 m.), the mean BMR was calculated as 1440 kcals. and the activity index as 1.9 (lower than that for women), giving a daily energy requirement of 2737 kcals.

This is close to the ICMR figure, and the ratio of male : female daily energy requirement of 81.6% (i.e. 2234/2737) is nearly identical to the ICMR suggested ratio of 0.82. In a detailed study of energy intake, expenditure and activity among men and women in Tamil Nadu, McNeill calculated the energy requirement of a rural subsistence farmer of average weight in her study area (50.9 kg.) as being 2858 kcals., using the FAO/WHO/UNU method. For these reasons, the ICMR consumption unit coefficients above were felt to suffice for the purposes of this study.

APPENDIX III

DERIVATION OF THE LOCAL POVERTY LINE

The local poverty line used in the household classification, was based on a weighted basket of the aggregation of production, plus purchases, minus sales of the most commonly consumed foods in the three main food categories i.e. rice, redgram and cooking oil. Thus, the percentage 'weights' of the three foodstuffs in the food index were calculated and are shown below, along with the calculation of the cost of the weighted food basket, sufficient for the daily calorie needs of one adult-equivalent (or consumption unit (CU)):

Weights in food index :	Rice	77.9%
	Redgram	13.4%
	Oil	8.7%

Food	Mean price per kg.(Rs.)	Cost per 100g.(Rs.)	kcals. per 100g(dry*)	Cost per 100 kcals.	Weighted cost(Rs.)
Rice	2.2	0.22	399*	0.055	0.043
Redgram	6.0	0.60	387*	0.155	0.021
Oil	16.0	1.60	900	0.180	0.016
				Total :	0.080

100 kcals. weighted basket costs : Rs. 0.080

2800 kcals. (1 CU) per day costs : Rs. 2.240

Cost per CU per year : Rs. 817.6

APPENDIX IV

CALCULATING A LORENZ CURVE AND GINI COEFFICIENT

The Gini Coefficient is a relatively sensitive measure of inequality. It is defined as half the average of the absolute differences in a continuous variable such income or asset value, between all possible pairs of individual units in the population considered i.e. all the differences being taken with a positive sign only.

An operational formula for the Gini Coefficient is :

$$G = \frac{2}{n^2 y} \sum_{i=1}^{n} {}^i y_i - \frac{n+1}{n}$$

where n = population size
y = mean income in the population
${}^i y_i$= income of the i th individual arranged in ascending order of magnitude.

The Gini coefficient lends itself to a graphical representation known as the Lorenz curve of concentration, which gives a picture of concentration of income shares at different percentile points of the distribution, thereby enabling both spatial and temporal comparisons.

In the graphical representation, twice the area between the curve and the line of equal distribution (i.e. the shaded area) represents the Gini coefficient (see Figure 3.5)

Method for calculating the Lorenz curve

i) Group data in ascending order of magnitude of income or land.

ii) Express the number of individuals in each group as a percentage of the total population and cumulate the percentages.

iii) Express the total area or income in each group as a percentage of the total area or income and cumulate the percentages.

iv) Plot the cumulative percentages of individuals against the cumulative percentage of land or income.

v) Draw the Lorenz curve.

vi) Calculate the percentage of land or income controlled by each decile and cumulate the percentages.

vii) Pair the cumulative percentages of land or income controlled by each decile.

viii) Multiply the pairs calculated in (7) by the decile of land or income controllers.

ix) $G = \dfrac{1000 - \text{total of (8)}}{1000}$

APPENDIX V

DEMOGRAPHIC DIFFERENTIATION

The Russian economist, A.V. Chayanov, argued that 'differentiation' amongst a homogeneous peasantry is brought about by cyclical processes, so that there is no long-term developing trend of polarisation of classes. He termed this 'demographic differentiation', according to which, the volume of the farm's activity expands and contracts with the development of the family cycle (represented by the ratio of earners to dependents within the household).

For Lenin, the differentiation of the peasantry and the process of capitalist development were identical (Rahman, 1986). Chayanov attempted to show that most of what Lenin took as evidence of class differentiation, could be interpreted as demographic differentiation.

In this study, controlling for family size, the Gini coefficient for total household income per CU was less than that for total household income, indicating some degree of life cycle effect on income inequality. However, this does not occur with assets; the two coefficients being virtually equal.

To determine whether demographic structure of the household affects work, output or operational landholding size, the ratio in the household of dependent CU/earner CU was regressed against the following variables :

Demographic structure significantly affected the household labour force participation, although in a non-Chayanovian manner. Here, as the ratio of dependents to earners in a household increased, it was the mean number of wage, not own, labour days that increased, giving rise to a statistically significant correlation between mean monthly total days work and this ratio. These were not ideal Chayanovian peasant farms from which the very principle of wage labour is excluded. Here, adults in families with high dependency ratios were more likely to hire themselves out as wage agricultural labourers to supplement income. As the ratio of dependents to earners increased, it was income from agricultural labour that increased significantly, not the value of agricultural output per acre of standardised landholding.

DEPENDENT VARIABLE	CORRELATION COEFFICIENT (r)
Mean monthly total (male and female) days worked	0.34 **
Mean monthly wage (male and female) days worked	0.24
Mean monthly own (male and female) days worked	0.01
Standardised operational landholding size	0.04
Total household asset value	0.02
Total household income	0.00
Total household value of produce	0.13
Total value of produce per own standardised acre	0.17
Mean adult individual income from agricultural labour	0.35 **

LEGEND : ** P<0.01

Chayanov's theory may have worked well enough for late 19th century Russia, where land was plentiful and not subject to clear property rights, but it cannot explain land and wealth variations in tribal Telengana.

INDEX